Tangled Desires:

Exploring the Intersection of BDSM and Psychology

Table of Contents

Introduction i

Overview ii

Chapter 1 1

Introduction to BDSM and Mental Health *1*
   Understanding BDSM and its Impact on Mental Health 2
   The importance of exploring the connection between BDSM and mental health 3

Chapter 2 6

Healthy Dynamics in BDSM Relationships *6*
   The role of communication and consent in BDSM 8
   Understanding power dynamics in BDSM relationships 9
   The importance of mutual respect and trust in BDSM relationships 11

Chapter 3 14

Trauma and BDSM *14*
   Understanding the potential impact of trauma on BDSM experiences 16
   Strategies for navigating trauma in BDSM contexts 18

Chapter 4 22

Dissociation in BDSM: Understanding the Psychological Impacts and Coping Mechanisms *22*
   What is Disassociation in BDSM? 23
   The psychology behind dissociation in BDSM 24
   The potential impacts of dissociation in BDSM 26
   Coping mechanisms for dissociation in BDSM 28

Chapter 5 31

Pitfalls and Misconceptions in BDSM *31*
   Addressing misconceptions of BDSM and mental health 33
   The dangers of engaging in BDSM without proper education and preparation 37
     The risks of physical injuries 39
     The risks of psychological harm 42
     The importance of understanding power dynamics and aftercare 43
   Navigating the stigma around BDSM and mental health 47

Chapter 6 49

The Intersection of Psychology and BDSM *49*
   The role of psychology in BDSM experiences 50
   How to approach BDSM through a psychological lens 51

Chapter 7 54

Cultivating Healthy BDSM Practices *54*
   Strategies for fostering a healthy BDSM practice 56
   Tips for building a positive BDSM community 58
   Balancing BDSM with other aspects of life 60

Chapter 8...**63**

Bringing it All Together...*63*
    Reflecting on the importance of healthy BDSM practices for mental health...65
    Encouragement to continue exploring the connection between BDSM and mental health 65

References **68**

About the Author...**73**

Introduction

BDSM has been widely misunderstood, and often misrepresented, in popular culture. This misrepresentation has contributed to the stigma surrounding BDSM and the assumption that it is harmful to mental health. However, the reality is that BDSM can be a healthy and fulfilling lifestyle, with the potential to enhance mental well-being when practiced responsibly.

This book is designed to provide insight and guidance for individuals who are interested in BDSM as a lifestyle and its impact on mental health. The aim of this book is to explore the connection between BDSM and mental health, focusing on healthier dynamics, effort in relationships, responsibility of each person, trauma and BDSM, and the pitfalls when we do not commit to the lifestyle. By addressing these topics, I hope to provide readers with the necessary knowledge and tools to engage in BDSM practices in a way that is safe, responsible, and fulfilling.

In this book, I will delve into the psychological and emotional aspects of BDSM, as well as the cultural and historical context of the lifestyle. We will explore the myths and misconceptions surrounding BDSM and mental health, and provide practical tips for practicing BDSM in a way that promotes mental and emotional well-being. We will also discuss the importance of communication, trust, and boundaries in BDSM relationships, and the potential consequences of ignoring these essential components.

Ultimately, this book is for anyone who wants to explore the intersection of BDSM and mental health in a responsible and fulfilling way. I hope that people will come away from this book with a better understanding of the benefits and potential pitfalls of BDSM, as well as practical tools for engaging in this lifestyle in a healthy and fulfilling way.

Overview

The intersection between BDSM and mental health is complex and multifaceted. On the one hand, BDSM can be a powerful tool for exploring and expressing our desires and emotions, helping us to build intimacy and trust in our relationships. However, engaging in BDSM can also be challenging, particularly when it comes to issues of communication, consent, and emotional safety. In this book, we will explore the different ways in which BDSM and mental health intersect, examining the potential risks and benefits of engaging in BDSM, and providing practical advice for creating healthy and responsible BDSM relationships.

One of the key themes that we will explore in this book is the importance of communication and consent in BDSM relationships. We will discuss the different ways in which power dynamics play out in BDSM relationships, and examine the ways in which trauma can impact our experiences of BDSM. By exploring these issues in depth, I hope to provide readers with a greater understanding of the risks and challenges of engaging in BDSM, and help them to build stronger, more fulfilling relationships with their partners.

Finally, we will examine the concept of responsibility in BDSM relationships, both in terms of taking care of our own emotional and physical needs, and in terms of being responsible to our partners. We will discuss the importance of setting clear boundaries, practicing self-care, and engaging in ongoing communication to ensure that our BDSM experiences are positive and fulfilling. By focusing on these themes, I hope to provide readers with a comprehensive overview of the intersection between BDSM and mental health, and equip them with the knowledge and tools they need to create healthy, responsible, and fulfilling BDSM relationships.

Chapter 1

Introduction to BDSM and Mental Health

BDSM, short for bondage and discipline, dominance and submission, and sadism and masochism, is a term used to describe a variety of sexual practices that involve consensual power exchange between partners. BDSM has become more visible in recent years, with media depictions and increased awareness leading to a greater understanding of the lifestyle. However, there is still a lack of understanding and education around BDSM, particularly in its connection to mental health.

Research has shown that BDSM can have both positive and negative effects on mental health. On the one hand, individuals who engage in BDSM report feeling more intimacy, trust, and emotional closeness with their partners, as well as increased feelings of empowerment and self-esteem (Connolly et al., 2006; Cross & Matheson, 2006). On the other hand, BDSM can also be associated with increased rates of anxiety, depression, and post-traumatic stress disorder, particularly among individuals who have experienced trauma (Moser & Kleinplatz, 2006; Sagarin et al., 2008).

Given the potential impact of BDSM on mental health, it is important to explore the connection between the two and understand the factors that contribute to healthier versus riskier BDSM practices. This chapter will provide an overview of BDSM and its impact on mental health, with a focus on the importance of exploring the connection between the two. We will examine both the positive and negative effects of BDSM on mental health, as well as the factors that contribute to healthier BDSM practices. Through this exploration, I hope to increase awareness and understanding of the intersection of BDSM and mental health, and promote healthier, safer BDSM practices for all involved.

Understanding BDSM and its impact on mental health

BDSM, or Bondage and Discipline, Dominance and Submission, Sadism and Masochism, is a consensual form of sexual expression and an umbrella term for various kinks and fetishes that involve power exchange, pain, and restraint (Wismeijer & van Assen, 2013). The practice of BDSM has long been stigmatized and misunderstood, with many people associating it with violence and abuse, even though BDSM is consensual and emphasizes safety and communication (Moser & Kleinplatz, 2006).

Research on the psychological impact of BDSM on mental health is still in its early stages, with much of it focused on dispelling myths and stereotypes surrounding BDSM. Studies have found that people who engage in BDSM activities have higher levels of mindfulness, openness to new experiences, and self-esteem than those who do not (Connolly et al., 2006; Cross & Matheson, 2006). BDSM activities have also been found to have stress-relieving effects, leading to increased feelings of well-being and relaxation (Sagarin et al., 2008).

One study examining the relationship between BDSM and mental health found that BDSM practitioners reported lower levels of psychological distress, anxiety, and depression than non-BDSM practitioners (Wismeijer & van Assen, 2013). Another study found that BDSM activities could be a coping mechanism for people with mental health issues such as anxiety, depression, and post-traumatic stress disorder (PTSD) (Kleinplatz & Moser, 2004).

While the research on BDSM and mental health is limited, the studies conducted so far suggest that BDSM can have a positive impact on mental health, providing stress relief, increased self-esteem, and a sense of community for those who engage in it. However, it is important to note that like any sexual activity, BDSM can have risks and should be practiced with informed consent, communication, and safety precautions in place.

Although there is a growing body of research exploring the impact of BDSM on mental health, more studies are needed to fully understand this complex relationship. For example, a study by Sagarin et al. (2008) found that individuals in BDSM relationships reported higher levels of relationship satisfaction and lower levels of psychological distress compared to those in non-BDSM relationships.

However, it is also important to note that some individuals who engage in BDSM may be at increased risk for certain mental health concerns. For example, individuals who have experienced past trauma or abuse may be more vulnerable to negative outcomes related to BDSM play. Additionally, there is some evidence to suggest that individuals who engage in certain BDSM practices, such as breath play or suspension, may be at increased risk for physical harm and injury.

BDSM is a consensual sexual practice that has been unfairly stigmatized and associated with violence and abuse. While research on the psychological impact of BDSM on mental health is still ongoing, early studies suggest that it can have positive effects, such as stress relief and increased self-esteem. However, to reap these benefits, it is essential to engage in BDSM safely and consensually. Mental health professionals should be knowledgeable about BDSM practices and potential risks when working with clients who engage in these activities, and individuals should educate themselves and their partners, communicate openly, and take appropriate safety measures. By promoting safe and healthy exploration of BDSM, we can help individuals experience sexual expression and intimacy in a fulfilling and positive way.

The importance of exploring the connection between BDSM and mental health

While research on the impact of BDSM on mental health is evolving, studies have suggested a complex relationship between the two. BDSM practitioners often report that engaging in BDSM activities has positive effects on their mental well-being, such as increased self-esteem, decreased anxiety and depression, and feelings of connection and community (Connolly et al., 2006; Cross & Matheson, 2006; Wismeijer & van Assen, 2013).

Furthermore, BDSM has been found to be a coping mechanism for people with mental health issues such as anxiety, depression, and PTSD, allowing them to reclaim power and control in a consensual and safe environment (Kleinplatz & Moser, 2004). Research has also shown that people who engage in BDSM tend to be more mindful and present in their daily lives, which may contribute to improved mental health outcomes (Wismeijer & van Assen, 2013).

However, it is important to note that some individuals who engage in BDSM may be at increased risk for certain mental health concerns. For example, research has found that individuals who have experienced past trauma or abuse may be more vulnerable to negative outcomes related to BDSM play (Richters et al., 2008). Additionally, certain BDSM practices, such as breath play or suspension, may carry a higher risk of physical harm or injury, which can have negative psychological consequences (Weinberg et al. 1984).

Despite the positive outcomes associated with BDSM play, there are still concerns that individuals who engage in BDSM may be at risk for certain mental health issues. For instance, a study found that individuals who engaged in BDSM had higher levels of posttraumatic stress disorder (PTSD) symptoms compared to non-BDSM practitioners, although this difference was not statistically significant (Richters et al., 2008). Additionally, another study found that individuals who engaged in BDSM were more likely to have borderline personality disorder (BPD) traits, which are characterized by emotional instability and difficulties with interpersonal relationships (Klement et al., 2016). We must keep in mind that studies are limited in their scope and may not necessarily reflect the experiences of all individuals who engage in BDSM.

Another area of concern when it comes to BDSM and mental health is the potential for harm and injury. BDSM activities such as impact play, knife play, and breath play, to name a few, have been found to be associated with physical harm and injury (Wismeijer & van Assen, 2013). In some cases, individuals may not be aware of the potential risks associated with certain BDSM practices or may not take appropriate safety precautions, which can lead to serious injury. It is important for individuals who engage in BDSM to educate themselves about the risks and to take appropriate safety measures to protect themselves and their partners. Mental health professionals should also be knowledgeable about the potential risks associated with BDSM play and be able to provide guidance and support to individuals who engage in these activities.

Studies have also explored the relationship between BDSM and trauma. Some researchers suggest that BDSM activities can be a coping mechanism for individuals who have experienced trauma, allowing them to reframe and regain control over past experiences (Waters & Galupo, 2019). In contrast, other studies have found that BDSM activities can be triggering for individuals with a history of trauma, potentially exacerbating symptoms and causing distress (New et al., 2021). It is important to note that engaging in BDSM activities after experiencing trauma should be approached with caution and only done with the guidance of a mental health professional.

Research has explored the ways in which BDSM can intersect with spirituality and provide individuals with a sense of psychological meaning and purpose (Baker, 2016). In her study, Baker (2016) found that some individuals engaged in what she termed "sacred kink," which involved BDSM activities with a spiritual or religious context. These individuals reported experiencing feelings of transcendence, connection, and personal growth as a result of their BDSM practices. For some, the experience of BDSM was seen to connect with a higher power or to explore existential questions. While not all individuals who engage in BDSM may experience it as a spiritual or meaningful practice, these findings suggest that for some, BDSM can have a positive impact on mental health and well-being. It is important for mental health professionals to be aware of the potential benefits of BDSM and to approach the topic with an open and non-judgmental attitude.

Overall, the relationship between BDSM and mental health is complex and multifaceted. While BDSM can have positive effects on mental well-being for some individuals, it is important to practice BDSM safely, with informed consent, communication, and safety measures in place. Mental health professionals should also be knowledgeable about BDSM practices and potential risks when working with clients who engage in these activities, and individuals should educate themselves and their partners to promote safe and healthy exploration of BDSM.

Chapter 2

Healthy Dynamics in BDSM Relationships

BDSM relationships can be complex and require a lot of communication and trust between partners to be healthy. In healthy BDSM relationships, all parties involved understand and have consented to the activities taking place. This means that all parties are fully aware of the risks and benefits of the activities and have agreed to participate willingly. Communication is essential to ensure that all parties understand each other's boundaries and that these boundaries are respected.

Trust is another critical component of healthy BDSM relationships. All parties should be able to trust that their partners will act in their best interests and respect their boundaries. This includes trust that the activities will not cause physical or emotional harm and that any limits or safe words will be respected. When trust is present, it allows all parties to feel safe and supported, which enhances the overall experience.

Additionally, healthy BDSM relationships prioritize the physical and emotional safety of all parties involved. This means that activities are planned with safety in mind, and measures are taken to minimize the risk of physical harm. Emotional safety is also essential, and partners should be aware of each other's emotional needs and boundaries.

Finally, healthy BDSM relationships are founded on mutual respect and a deep understanding of each other's needs and desires. All parties should feel valued and appreciated, and their unique preferences and boundaries should be respected. This includes respecting each other's privacy and maintaining confidentiality about the activities taking place.

In summary, healthy BDSM relationships are based on communication, trust, physical and emotional safety, mutual respect, and understanding. By prioritizing these elements, partners can create a fulfilling and enjoyable BDSM experience that meets the needs of all parties involved.

The role of communication and consent in BDSM

Consent is a central tenet of BDSM dynamics and is often seen as more important than in vanilla or normal relationships. Communication is key in both types of relationships, but in BDSM dynamics, it takes on a heightened significance. Bloomer (2019) explains that in BDSM, consent is negotiated and ongoing, with partners discussing and agreeing on activities before engaging in them. This negotiation process can involve discussing specific acts, boundaries, and any limitations, as well as establishing safe words and checking in throughout the activity.

Yost and Hunter (2012) discuss how communication and consent in BDSM dynamics can evolve as partners become more comfortable with each other and develop a deeper understanding of each other's needs and desires. However, the effort required to maintain communication and consent can be significant, as BDSM activities can involve physical and emotional risks.

The importance of consent in BDSM dynamics extends beyond the relationship itself. Klement et al. (2016) found that participating in a culture of consent, as seen in the BDSM community, was associated with lower rape-supportive beliefs. This highlights the positive impact of emphasizing the importance of consent not just within BDSM dynamics but in broader society as well.

Moreover, the validity of consent and communication in BDSM dynamics can also be seen in the way that it fosters a sense of agency and empowerment for the participants. By giving individuals the power to negotiate and establish their boundaries, as well as providing a safe environment to explore their desires, BDSM dynamics can provide a sense of control and agency that may be lacking in other areas of their lives. This can have positive effects on their self-esteem and overall well-being.

Additionally, the emphasis on communication and consent in BDSM dynamics can also create a deeper sense of trust and intimacy between partners. When partners can communicate openly and honestly about their desires and boundaries, they develop a deeper understanding of each other's needs and fears. This can lead to a greater sense of emotional intimacy and closeness in the relationship, as partners feel more comfortable being vulnerable with each other.

It is also worth noting that the emphasis on communication and consent in BDSM dynamics can help to dispel some of the myths and stereotypes surrounding BDSM practices. BDSM is often portrayed in the media as abusive or non-consensual, which can contribute to stigma and misunderstanding. By emphasizing the importance of consent and communication, the BDSM community can help to educate others and promote a more accurate understanding of the dynamics involved.

Finally, Fan and Han (2008) explored the neural mechanisms involved in empathy for pain in BDSM practitioners. They found that BDSM practitioners showed greater empathy for pain in others compared to non-practitioners. This suggests that BDSM dynamics, which prioritize communication and consent, may foster greater emotional awareness and empathy in individuals. Overall, the emphasis on communication and consent in BDSM dynamics highlights the importance of open and honest communication in all relationships. BDSM dynamics offer a unique framework for negotiating consent, which can serve as a model for broader society.

<u>Understanding power dynamics in BDSM relationships</u>

Power exchange is a crucial aspect of BDSM relationships that requires a deep understanding of the different types of power dynamics involved. Research has shown that BDSM activities can be psychologically beneficial for participants, but only if they are practiced safely, sanely, and consensually (Connolly et al., 2006).

Restricted compliance, limited ongoing consent, conditional submission, 24/7 lifestyle dynamics, and total power exchange are the main types of power exchange dynamics in BDSM relationships. Partners should discuss and agree on the type of power exchange they want to participate in before engaging in any BDSM activities. This coupled, with ongoing personal research and understanding into the roles one chooses to identify in, as well as all of what that encompasses.

According to Ramey (2013), restricted compliance is a good starting point for people who are new to BDSM and want to explore power dynamics. Limited ongoing consent requires more commitment from both partners and can involve multiple BDSM sessions. Conditional submission involves greater control given to the Dominant partner and can include more risky or emotionally intense activities. 24/7 lifestyle dynamics require a high level of commitment and trust from both partners and can involve a variety of BDSM activities outside of the bedroom. Total power exchange is the most intense of all BDSM dynamics and requires a soaring level of trust and communication to engage in it safely.

The covenants of power exchange and authority transfer are based on three key principles: compliance, relinquishment, and subservience (Baker, 2019). Compliance involves following the commands of authority, leading to a change in behavior. Relinquishment is an act of submitting oneself into the possession of another, letting go of control. Subservience is the state of being under the control of someone else and serving them. A covenant signifies deep emotional ties and is more than an agreement; it is an enduring promise, a state of being in the relationship and not just acts of doing (Baumeister, 1988).

It is important to note that BDSM activities rely on the explicit and ongoing consent of all parties involved. The dominant partner has a responsibility to ensure the safety and well-being of the submissive partner throughout the interaction. Both partners must discuss specific activities, limits, and boundaries and establish safe words and other communication tools to ensure that the BDSM activities are safe, consensual, and enjoyable for all parties involved.

While the idea of power exchange may sound intimidating to some, it can be a deeply fulfilling experience for those who engage in it. Studies have shown that BDSM activities, including power exchange, can lead to increased emotional and sexual intimacy, communication, and relationship satisfaction among participants (Wismeijer & van Assen, 2013).

Furthermore, BDSM activities, including power exchange, are not inherently abusive or harmful. In fact, research has shown that BDSM practitioners often have lower levels of psychological distress and higher levels of well-being and rejection sensitivity compared to non-practitioners (Sagarin et al., 2008).

However, it is important to note that BDSM activities, including power exchange, can still pose physical and emotional risks if not practiced safely and with consent. Therefore, it is crucial for partners to establish clear boundaries and safe words from the onset, to ensure that both parties are comfortable and safe during the interaction (Kolmes et al.2006).

Additionally, seeking out education and resources on BDSM and power dynamics can help partners better understand the nuances of power exchange and engage in it more safely and confidently. Some resources include online forums and communities, workshops, and books on BDSM and power dynamics (Weiss, 2006).

Through this understanding we realize, power exchange is a crucial aspect of BDSM relationships, and understanding the various types of power exchange dynamics is essential for safe and fulfilling experiences. It is important for partners to communicate effectively and establish clear boundaries and safe words to ensure safety and well-being during the interaction. Seeking out education and resources on BDSM and power dynamics can also help partners engage in power exchange more safely and confidently.

The importance of mutual respect and trust in BDSM relationships

BDSM relationships, like any other intimate relationships, require a foundation of mutual respect and trust. In fact, these values are even more crucial in BDSM relationships, where partners engage in activities that involve power dynamics and potential risks. Without trust and respect, BDSM activities can quickly become dangerous and damaging to both partners.

Respect is the foundation of any healthy relationship, including BDSM relationships. In a BDSM relationship, the dominant partner must respect the submissive partner's limits, boundaries, and wishes. This means that the dominant partner must refrain from engaging in activities that the submissive partner is uncomfortable with, and must always prioritize their safety and well-being. Similarly, the submissive partner must respect the dominant partner's desires and limits, and must also communicate openly and honestly with their partner about their needs and boundaries.

Trust is another essential element of a healthy BDSM relationship. Both partners must trust each other to engage in BDSM activities safely, sanely, and consensually. Trust is built through open and honest communication, consistent follow-through on commitments, and a willingness to listen to and respect each other's needs and desires. In a BDSM relationship, trust can also involve the submissive partner placing a great deal of trust in the dominant partner's ability to keep them safe and provide for their well-being.

Research has shown that BDSM activities, including power exchange dynamics, can be psychologically beneficial for participants when they are practiced safely and consensually (Connolly et al., 2006). However, in order to engage in these activities safely, trust and respect are crucial, and become the fundamental building block to the dynamic over time. Without these values, BDSM activities can quickly become abusive and traumatic.

BDSM activities can also be deeply intimate and emotionally fulfilling for both partners when practiced with respect and trust. The power dynamics involved in BDSM activities can create a sense of vulnerability and openness that can lead to greater emotional intimacy and connection between partners. In fact, some research has suggested that BDSM practitioners may experience greater relationship satisfaction and communication compared to non-practitioners, in areas of happiness, well-being and stability. (Wismeijer & van Assen, 2013).

However, in order to achieve these benefits, both partners must be willing to prioritize mutual respect and trust. This means communicating openly and honestly about desires, boundaries, and limits, and being willing to listen to and respect each other's needs. It also means being willing to stop or modify activities if one partner becomes uncomfortable or feels unsafe, and establishing clear safe words and communication tools to ensure that BDSM activities are consensual and safe. Listening and building a rapport over time, without rushing either through the process.

Mutual respect and trust are vital essentials in any healthy BDSM relationship. These values allow partners to engage in BDSM activities safely, consensually, and with the understanding that the other person's well-being is of the utmost importance. BDSM, when practiced in this way, can provide a deeply intimate and satisfying experience for both partners, enhancing their emotional connection and overall relationship satisfaction. To achieve this, it is essential that both partners communicate openly and honestly, setting clear boundaries and expectations for their BDSM activities. By prioritizing mutual respect and trust, BDSM can be a healthy and fulfilling part of a couple's sexual and emotional life.

Chapter 3

Trauma and BDSM

One of the most important factors to consider when exploring the relationship between trauma and BDSM is the impact of early life experiences. Childhood trauma, such as physical, emotional, or sexual abuse, can have a profound impact on an individual's psychological development and can shape their relationship with power and control in adulthood. Research has shown that individuals who have experienced childhood trauma may be more likely to engage in BDSM activities as a way of processing and coping with past experiences of abuse (Brown et al., 2016).

Furthermore, it is important to note that not all BDSM activities are the same, and some may be more likely to trigger traumatic responses than others. For example, certain activities may be associated with a higher risk of physical injury or emotional distress, such as those that involve asphyxiation or intense pain. It is important for individuals who engage in BDSM activities to be aware of these risks and to communicate openly with their partner about their boundaries and limitations in order to ensure a safe and consensual experience.

At the same time, it is important to recognize that BDSM activities can also be a source of healing and growth for individuals who have experienced trauma. Studies have shown that engaging in consensual BDSM activities can help individuals to build trust, increase communication, and develop a sense of mastery and control over their own bodies and experiences (Kleinplatz & Moser, 2006).

However, it is imperative for individuals to approach BDSM activities in a thoughtful and intentional way, particularly if they have a history of trauma. This may involve seeking out professional counseling or therapy to process past experiences and develop healthy coping mechanisms. It is also important to prioritize safety and communication in BDSM activities, and to be aware of the potential risks and consequences of engaging in certain activities.

Ultimately, the relationship between trauma and BDSM is complex and multifaceted, and requires a nuanced understanding of the factors that contribute to individual experiences. By approaching BDSM activities with respect, intentionality, and an awareness of potential risks and benefits, individuals can engage in consensual and fulfilling experiences that promote healing, growth, and connection.

Understanding the potential impact of trauma on BDSM experiences

The potential impact of trauma on BDSM experiences is a complex and multifaceted issue that requires a deep understanding of the psychological, emotional, and physical effects of traumatic experiences. Trauma can take many forms, including childhood abuse, sexual assault, and combat-related trauma, among others, and can have a profound impact on an individual's perception of power, control, and trust. As such, it is crucial to approach BDSM activities with sensitivity and care, particularly when individuals have a history of trauma.

One of the most significant ways in which trauma can impact BDSM experiences is through the development of triggers. Triggers are specific stimuli that can elicit intense emotional or physical reactions in individuals who have experienced trauma, and can include anything from certain words or phrases to specific types of touch. These triggers can be particularly challenging in BDSM contexts, where activities may involve power dynamics, physical restraint, or other potentially triggering elements. It is therefore essential for individuals to communicate openly and honestly with their partners about their triggers and to establish clear boundaries and safe words to ensure a safe and consensual experience (Moser, 2010).

Another potential impact of trauma on BDSM experiences is the development of dissociation. Dissociation is a coping mechanism that involves detaching oneself from their surroundings or experiences to avoid overwhelming emotional or physical pain. Individuals who have experienced trauma may be more prone to dissociative experiences during BDSM activities, particularly if the activities involve elements that may be reminiscent of past traumatic experiences. This can be particularly challenging for individuals who are seeking to engage in BDSM activities to process and heal from past traumas, as dissociation can hinder the ability to connect with one's body and emotions (Steele & van der Hart, 2015).

However, it is important to note that BDSM activities can also be a powerful tool for healing and growth for individuals who have experienced trauma. BDSM activities that prioritize communication, trust, and consent can help individuals to develop a sense of agency and control over their bodies and experiences, which can be empowering for those who have experienced trauma-related powerlessness (Hawkins & O'Hare, 2017). Additionally, BDSM activities can facilitate the development of strong emotional connections with partners, which can be particularly meaningful for individuals who have experienced past relationship trauma (Hébert & Weaver, 2014).

To maximize the potential benefits of BDSM activities for individuals who have experienced trauma, it is essential to approach these activities in a thoughtful and intentional way. This may involve seeking out professional counseling or therapy to process past experiences and develop healthy coping mechanisms. It is also crucial to prioritize communication, trust, and consent in BDSM activities, and to be aware of the potential risks and consequences of engaging in certain activities. This includes understanding the potential physical and emotional risks associated with activities such as asphyxiation, intense pain, or bondage, and establishing clear boundaries and safe words with partners to ensure a safe and consensual experience (Weinberg et al., 1984).

In addition to prioritizing safety and communication, it is also essential to recognize the importance of aftercare in BDSM activities. Aftercare involves taking care of oneself and one's partner emotionally and physically following BDSM activities, which can include activities such as cuddling, affirmations, or simply checking in with one another. For individuals who have experienced trauma, aftercare can be particularly important to re-establish feelings of safety and trust following potentially triggering experiences (Dancer et. al, 2006).

Overall, understanding the potential impact of trauma on BDSM experiences requires a nuanced and multifaceted approach. While trauma can shape an individual's attitudes towards power, control, and sexuality, it is important to recognize that BDSM activities can also be a source of healing and growth for those who have experienced trauma. Practitioners of BDSM should prioritize communication, consent, and safety, and individuals who have experienced trauma should approach BDSM activities in a thoughtful and intentional way, potentially seeking professional counselling or therapy to process past experiences and develop healthy coping mechanisms. By taking these precautions, individuals can engage in BDSM activities in a safe and consensual manner, while also potentially finding healing and growth in their experiences.

Strategies for navigating trauma in BDSM contexts

Trauma is a ubiquitous and deeply personal experience that can have lasting effects on an individual's psyche and behavior. For some, the exploration of BDSM activities can be a means of processing and overcoming past traumatic experiences. However, the inherent power dynamics and physicality of BDSM activities can also pose unique challenges and risks for those who have experienced trauma. Therefore, it is essential for individuals who engage in BDSM activities to understand and implement effective strategies for navigating trauma in BDSM contexts.

One key strategy for navigating trauma in BDSM contexts is the development of a strong sense of self-awareness. This involves taking the time to reflect on one's past experiences and how they may impact one's current attitudes towards power, control, and sexuality. It also involves recognizing and understanding one's triggers and establishing clear boundaries with partners to avoid potentially triggering situations. Research has shown that individuals who engage in BDSM activities with a strong sense of self-awareness are more likely to experience positive outcomes and avoid negative consequences (Hébert & Weaver, 2014).

Another crucial strategy for navigating trauma in BDSM contexts is the prioritization of communication and consent. This involves openly discussing one's boundaries, desires, and expectations with partners, as well as ensuring that all activities are safe, sane, and consensual. Effective communication and consent can help to foster a sense of trust and mutual respect between partners, which can be particularly important for individuals who have experienced trauma-related powerlessness. Studies have shown that individuals who engage in BDSM activities with a focus on communication and consent are more likely to report positive emotional experiences and relationship satisfaction (Hawkins & O'Hare, 2017).

Identifying trauma triggers is a crucial step in developing effective strategies for navigating BDSM activities in a safe and healthy manner. Trauma triggers are specific stimuli or situations that can trigger negative emotional and physical responses in individuals who have experienced trauma. These triggers can be highly personal and may vary from person to person, making it essential for individuals to identify and communicate their triggers with their partners.

Some common trauma triggers in BDSM contexts include physical restraints, humiliation, and the use of certain words or phrases. However, triggers can also be more subtle and may be related to the specific circumstances or context in which BDSM activities are taking place. For example, being in a particular room or being with a certain partner may trigger memories or emotions related to past traumatic experiences.

To effectively identify and communicate trauma triggers, individuals must first develop a strong sense of self-awareness. This involves taking the time to reflect on one's past experiences and identifying patterns of behavior or situations that have been triggering in the past. It also involves recognizing and understanding one's emotional and physical responses to potential triggers.

Once individuals have identified their trauma triggers, it is essential to communicate them clearly and effectively with partners. This can involve having a frank and open discussion about past experiences and triggers, as well as establishing clear boundaries and safe words to ensure that partners are aware of potential triggers and can take steps to avoid them. Effective communication and consent can help to foster a sense of trust and mutual respect between partners, which can be particularly important for individuals who have experienced trauma-related powerlessness.

In addition to identifying and communicating trauma triggers, it is also important to develop strategies for coping with triggers if they do occur during BDSM activities. This can involve techniques such as grounding exercises, deep breathing, or visualization, as well as taking breaks or slowing down the pace of activities. It may also involve establishing a clear plan for aftercare, which involves providing emotional and physical support to partners after BDSM activities have concluded.

Overall, identifying trauma triggers is a crucial step in developing effective strategies for navigating BDSM activities in a safe and healthy manner. By developing a strong sense of self-awareness, communicating clearly with partners, and developing coping strategies, individuals can engage in BDSM activities in a way that is empowering and healing rather than retraumatizing.

Coping with regression during BDSM activities is a crucial component of navigating trauma triggers and ensuring that activities remain safe and healthy. Regression, which refers to a return to childlike behaviors or thought patterns, can occur when individuals are triggered by past traumatic experiences during BDSM play. It is important for individuals to have effective coping mechanisms in place to deal with regression, as this can help to prevent retraumatization and ensure a positive and empowering experience.

One effective coping mechanism for dealing with regression during BDSM activities is grounding exercises. Grounding exercises involve focusing on the present moment and physical sensations in order to help individuals stay connected to reality and prevent feelings of overwhelm. This can involve techniques such as deep breathing, visualization, or focusing on physical sensations such as the feeling of the ground beneath one's feet. Research has shown that grounding exercises can be an effective way to reduce symptoms of anxiety and dissociation (Price et al., 2019).

Another effective coping mechanism for dealing with regression during BDSM activities is the use of safe words and clear boundaries. Establishing clear boundaries and using safe words can help individuals feel more in control of their experiences and can provide a sense of safety and security. In the event that regression does occur, safe words and clear boundaries can also be used to signal a need for a break or to stop activities altogether. This can help to prevent retraumatization and ensure that individuals are able to continue to engage in BDSM activities in a safe and healthy manner.

It is also important for individuals to have a clear plan for aftercare in place in the event that regression does occur during BDSM activities. Aftercare involves providing emotional and physical support to partners after BDSM activities have concluded, and can be particularly important for individuals who have experienced trauma-related powerlessness. Aftercare can involve activities such as cuddling, checking in with partners, or providing water and snacks. Research has shown that aftercare can be an important component of BDSM activities, as it can help to promote feelings of safety, connection, and trust (Pincus et al., 2018).

In summary, coping with regression during BDSM activities is an essential component of navigating trauma triggers and ensuring a positive and empowering experience. Grounding exercises, clear boundaries and safe words, and aftercare are all effective coping mechanisms that can help individuals to cope with regression and prevent retraumatization. By implementing these strategies and developing a strong sense of self-awareness, individuals can engage in BDSM activities in a way that is safe, healthy, and empowering.

Chapter 4

Dissociation in BDSM: Understanding the Psychological Impacts and Coping Mechanisms

BDSM, like any other sexual activity, can be accompanied by psychological responses, including dissociation. Dissociation is an altered state of consciousness that can be both positive and negative, but it is important to understand how it can impact individuals who engage in BDSM play. In this post, we will explore the psychology behind dissociation in BDSM, the potential impacts it can have, and coping mechanisms that can be used to minimize negative experiences.

Dissociation in BDSM can occur in various ways. For some individuals, it may involve detaching from the physical sensations of pain or pleasure. For others, it could mean dissociating from their thoughts or emotions, feeling as if they are watching the scene from outside their body. In some cases, dissociation can also be triggered by a past trauma or an overwhelming experience during BDSM play. Regardless of the cause, dissociation can affect one's ability to communicate their boundaries and preferences, leading to potential harm and trauma.

It is essential to note that dissociation is not always harmful, and many BDSM practitioners intentionally use dissociative techniques to enhance their experience. However, it is crucial to differentiate between a conscious choice to dissociate and an involuntary response to a trigger. By understanding the underlying psychological mechanisms and learning to recognize the signs of dissociation, individuals can engage in BDSM play safely and confidently, without compromising their mental and emotional wellbeing.

What is Disassociation in BDSM?

Dissociation is a psychological phenomenon where an individual experiences a sense of detachment from their physical or emotional state. In the context of BDSM play, dissociation can occur as a coping mechanism to manage the intense physical and psychological sensations that may arise during the activity. For example, a submissive partner may experience a sense of detachment from their physical sensations or surroundings to manage the intense sensations they may experience during bondage or impact play. Similarly, a dominant partner may dissociate as a means of compartmentalizing their feelings and emotions in order to maintain control and provide a safe and consensual experience for their submissive partner. While dissociation can be a natural response to the intensity of BDSM play, it is important to understand its potential impacts and how to manage it in a safe and consensual way.

It is important to note that dissociation can also occur involuntarily, triggered by past trauma or overwhelming emotions. In such cases, dissociation can be distressing and potentially harmful, as it can interfere with an individual's ability to communicate their needs and boundaries. It is crucial for BDSM practitioners to have a solid understanding of dissociation and its potential impacts to ensure that all parties involved feel safe, respected, and heard.

Some common signs of dissociation in BDSM include feeling disconnected from one's surroundings or body, experiencing a sense of numbness or detachment, and feeling as though one is watching the scene from outside of their body. If any of these signs are present during BDSM play, it is important to pause and check in with all parties involved to ensure that everyone feels safe and comfortable. Engaging in aftercare, such as cuddling, talking, or simply being present with each other, can also help to ground individuals and reduce the likelihood of negative impacts from dissociation.

There are different types of dissociation that can be experienced during BDSM play, each with unique characteristics and impacts. Some of these types include:

- Depersonalization: a sense of detachment from oneself, which can lead to feeling like an observer of one's own body and experiences.

- Derealization: a sense of detachment from one's surroundings, which can lead to feelings of unreality or disconnection from the external world.
- Dissociative amnesia: the inability to recall events or experiences that occurred during BDSM play, which may occur as a result of traumatic or overwhelming experiences.
- Trance states: a focused and altered state of consciousness that can be entered intentionally or spontaneously during BDSM play, which can enhance the intensity of the experience.

It is important to note that dissociation can have both positive and negative impacts, and individuals who engage in BDSM play should be aware of the potential risks associated with dissociation and how to minimize those risks.

Dissociation in BDSM can be a complex and multifaceted experience, and it is crucial to understand its potential impacts and how to manage it safely. As noted by Ruth Blizard in the article "Masochistic and Sadistic Ego States: Dissociative Solutions to the Dilemma of Attachment to an Abusive Caretaker" (2001), dissociation can be a solution to attachment to an abusive caregiver and can manifest as masochistic or sadistic ego states in BDSM play. However, it's important to recognize that dissociation can also be triggered by past trauma or overwhelming emotions, and it can interfere with an individual's ability to communicate their needs and boundaries. Practitioners of BDSM should prioritize open communication, enthusiastic consent, and aftercare to minimize the risks associated with dissociation and ensure that all parties involved feel safe and respected.

The psychology behind dissociation in BDSM

Dissociation during BDSM play is a complex phenomenon that has been studied by various researchers. Hillier's (2019) study on the impact of childhood trauma and personality on kinkiness in adulthood sheds light on the potential psychological factors that may contribute to dissociation during BDSM play. According to Hillier's (2019) research, individuals who have experienced childhood trauma may be more likely to engage in BDSM activities to cope with the trauma. Additionally, personality traits such as openness to experience and sensation-seeking have also been associated with kinkiness in adulthood, which may contribute to the appeal of BDSM play.

While BDSM play can be a consensual and enjoyable experience for many individuals, it is important to understand the potential risks and psychological factors that may contribute to dissociation during play. Hillier's (2019) research provides insight into the complex interplay between childhood trauma, personality, and kinkiness in adulthood, and highlights the need for further research on the topic.

There are several psychological factors that can contribute to dissociation during BDSM play. These include:

- Past trauma: Individuals who have experienced trauma in the past may be more likely to dissociate during BDSM play as a coping mechanism to manage intense emotions and sensations.
- Control and power dynamics: The power dynamic in BDSM relationships can create a sense of detachment from one's emotions and experiences as a way to maintain control and safety.
- Intense sensations: The intense physical and psychological sensations that can arise during BDSM play can overwhelm an individual's coping mechanisms, leading to dissociation.
- Context and setting: The environment in which BDSM play occurs can impact an individual's dissociative response. For example, feeling unsafe or uncomfortable in the setting can increase the likelihood of dissociation.

Understanding these psychological factors can help individuals who engage in BDSM play to identify potential triggers for dissociation and take steps to minimize the risk of negative experiences. By creating a safe and consensual environment, communicating openly with partners, and practicing aftercare, individuals can mitigate the risk of dissociation and promote a positive experience.

The power dynamic in BDSM relationships can create a unique context for dissociation to occur. In these relationships, individuals may assume roles of dominance or submission, which can impact their emotional and psychological state during play. For submissive partners, the act of relinquishing control to a dominant partner can be a source of emotional intensity, leading to dissociation as a way to manage these feelings. Alternatively, dominant partners may dissociate as a means of compartmentalizing their feelings and emotions in order to maintain control and provide a safe and consensual experience for their submissive partner. The power dynamic can create a sense of detachment from one's emotions and experiences, leading to dissociation as a coping mechanism. It's important for individuals in BDSM relationships to communicate openly about their desires, boundaries, and emotional state, and to practice aftercare to promote a positive and safe experience for all parties involved.

The potential impacts of dissociation in BDSM

BDSM can elicit a range of psychological and emotional responses, and dissociation is one of them. It can be experienced as a positive coping mechanism, helping individuals manage intense sensations and emotions during play. On the other hand, dissociation can also be experienced as a negative response, interfering with an individual's ability to fully engage with the experience and potentially leading to emotional distress. Therefore, understanding the potential impacts of dissociation in BDSM is crucial to ensuring a safe, consensual, and enjoyable experience.

The effects of dissociation can vary from person to person, and it is important to recognize that what might be a positive experience for one person could be negative for another. Some individuals may find dissociation to be a useful tool for managing difficult emotions, while others may find it to be disorienting and upsetting.

Regardless of individual responses, it is important to be aware of the potential impacts of dissociation in BDSM and to take steps to minimize the risks involved. Here are some differences between the two:

Positive impacts:
- Heightened sensations: Dissociation can allow individuals to experience heightened sensations and pleasure during BDSM play.

- Enhanced emotional regulation: For individuals who have experienced past trauma or struggle with emotional regulation, dissociation can be a helpful coping mechanism that allows them to manage intense emotions during BDSM play.

- Altered states of consciousness: Some individuals may intentionally enter a dissociative state as a way to explore altered states of consciousness and enhance their BDSM experience.

Negative impacts:

- Increased risk of injury: Dissociation can impact an individual's ability to accurately assess their physical and emotional state, potentially leading to an increased risk of injury during BDSM play.

- Emotional dysregulation: Dissociation can also impact an individual's ability to regulate their emotions after the BDSM play is over, potentially leading to negative emotional experiences or flashbacks.

- Disconnection from partner: If both partners are not aware of and consenting to dissociative experiences, it can lead to a sense of disconnection from each other and potentially damage the relationship.

While dissociation can have both positive and negative impacts on individuals during BDSM play, it is crucial to recognize that the experience is subjective and can vary greatly from person to person. Some individuals may find dissociation to be an essential component of their BDSM practice, while others may find it overwhelming or triggering. Therefore, it is vital to communicate openly with partners about personal preferences, boundaries, and potential triggers to ensure a safe and enjoyable experience for all parties involved.

Moreover, practicing safe and consensual BDSM play is crucial to minimize the potential negative impacts of dissociation. Establishing clear boundaries, utilizing safe words, and engaging in open communication with partners can help create a sense of safety and trust during BDSM play. It is also crucial to engage in self-care practices after BDSM play, such as seeking emotional support from trusted individuals or engaging in relaxing activities, to process any intense emotions or sensations that may arise. By prioritizing safety, trust, and open communication, individuals can minimize the risks associated with dissociation during BDSM play and cultivate a positive and empowering BDSM experience.

Coping mechanisms for dissociation in BDSM

Dissociation is a complex psychological response that can be experienced during BDSM play, and it is important for individuals engaging in BDSM to understand how to cope with dissociative experiences in a safe and consensual manner. Coping mechanisms for dissociation in BDSM can help individuals manage intense emotions and sensations and promote a positive experience. In this post, we will explore some practical coping mechanisms for dissociation in BDSM play and provide tips on how to communicate with partners and practice self-care to minimize the potential negative impacts of dissociation.

If you experience dissociative experiences during BDSM play, it is important to have coping mechanisms in place to manage intense emotions and sensations. Here are some practical tips on how to cope with dissociation during BDSM play:

- Establish a safe word or signal with your partner(s) to indicate when you need to stop or slow down.
- Use grounding techniques, such as focusing on your breath, to bring your attention back to the present moment.
- Communicate with your partner(s) about your needs and boundaries before and during BDSM play.
- Engage in aftercare activities, such as cuddling or talking with your partner(s), to promote feelings of safety and comfort.
- Practice self-care, such as taking a warm bath or engaging in gentle exercise, to help regulate your emotions after a BDSM session.
- Seek professional help if you are experiencing dissociation or other mental health concerns.

In addition to the coping mechanisms listed above, it may also be helpful to incorporate mindfulness practices, such as meditation or yoga, into your daily routine to promote overall mental well-being and resilience. It is also essential to engage in ongoing communication with your partner(s) about your experiences with dissociation and to seek support from mental health professionals if needed. Remember that prioritizing your mental and emotional well-being is a crucial aspect of engaging in safe, consensual, and fulfilling BDSM play.

Communication, trust, and aftercare are key components to minimizing the potential negative impacts of dissociation during BDSM play. Here are some ways in which they can help:

- Communication: Open and honest communication with your partner(s) is essential to ensure that everyone is on the same page and that boundaries are respected. It is important to discuss your needs and preferences before and during BDSM play, and to use clear and unambiguous signals to indicate when you need to stop or slow down.

- Trust: Developing trust with your partner(s) is essential to feel safe and secure during BDSM play. Trust can be built through communication, consistent behavior, and respecting boundaries. When trust is established, it can help individuals feel more comfortable exploring their desires and experiences, and can help minimize the risk of negative impacts.

- Aftercare: Aftercare involves activities that promote feelings of safety, comfort, and emotional support after BDSM play. Aftercare activities can include cuddling, talking, or engaging in gentle activities together. Aftercare can help individuals feel more connected to their partner(s) and can help them process intense emotions or sensations.

By prioritizing communication, trust, and aftercare, individuals can minimize the potential negative impacts of dissociation during BDSM play and can ensure a safe and consensual experience.

Dissociation is a complex psychological response that can occur during BDSM play, but it does not have to be a negative experience. By understanding the psychology behind dissociation and its potential impacts, individuals who engage in BDSM can take steps to minimize any potential negative effects and promote a safe and consensual experience. It's important to note that dissociation can be both positive and negative, depending on the individual's experience and coping mechanisms. While it may provide a sense of release and relaxation for some individuals, it can also lead to feelings of disconnection, fear, or anxiety for others.

Coping mechanisms such as grounding techniques, mindfulness, and breathing exercises can help individuals manage dissociative experiences during BDSM play. Additionally, prioritizing communication, trust, and aftercare can help minimize the potential negative impacts of dissociation and promote a positive experience. It's essential to have open and honest communication with your partner(s), establish trust, and engage in aftercare activities that promote feelings of safety, comfort, and emotional support.

By prioritizing and using coping mechanisms to manage dissociative experiences, individuals can enjoy a safe and consensual BDSM experience. These techniques not only benefit those affected by dissociation but also the BDSM community as a whole. Prioritizing open communication and trust can help to reduce stigma and create a more inclusive environment for all individuals to explore their sexuality and desires. Additionally, promoting aftercare activities that focus on emotional support and physical comfort can foster a sense of community and connectedness within the BDSM community. Ultimately, by prioritizing these key components, individuals can create a safe, consensual, and positive BDSM experience for themselves and their partners.

Chapter 5

Pitfalls and Misconceptions in BDSM

BDSM is a topic that has been met with a great deal of misunderstanding and stigma in society. Despite its growing popularity and acceptance, many people still hold misconceptions about what BDSM is, and how it relates to mental health. In this chapter, we will explore some of the most common pitfalls and misconceptions surrounding BDSM, and how they can impact mental health.

One of the most prevalent misconceptions about BDSM is that it is inherently abusive or pathological. This idea is often fueled by sensationalized media portrayals of BDSM that depict it as deviant and dangerous behavior. However, research has consistently shown that individuals who engage in consensual BDSM tend to be well-adjusted and mentally healthy. In fact, some studies have suggested that BDSM can have positive psychological benefits, such as increased intimacy, communication, and self-awareness.

Despite this evidence, there are still many who believe that BDSM is a sign of mental illness or trauma. This stigma can make it difficult for individuals who engage in BDSM to seek out help or support when they need it. It is important to recognize that BDSM is a valid and healthy form of sexual expression, and that individuals who practice it are not inherently damaged or disturbed.

However, it is also important to acknowledge that engaging in BDSM without proper education and preparation can be dangerous. BDSM activities can involve physical risks, such as choking, bondage, and impact play, as well as psychological risks, such as emotional triggers and trauma. In the next section, we will explore some of the dangers of engaging in BDSM without adequate knowledge and preparation, and how they can impact mental health.

By addressing some of the most common misconceptions about BDSM and mental health, as well as the dangers of engaging in BDSM without proper education and preparation, this chapter aims to shed light on the nuances of this complex and often misunderstood subculture. Additionally, we will explore the stigmas surrounding BDSM and mental health, and provide insights on how to navigate them. With a better understanding of the pitfalls and misconceptions in BDSM, we can work towards a more informed and accepting society that recognizes the value and legitimacy of BDSM as a form of sexual expression.

Addressing misconceptions of BDSM and mental health

In Chapter 3, we explored the complex relationship between BDSM and trauma, discussing how BDSM can be both a source of healing and a potential trigger for those with a history of trauma. We also emphasized the importance of safety and consent in BDSM activities, particularly for those who have experienced trauma.

In this area, we shift our focus to another important aspect of BDSM - its relationship with mental health. This subsection aims to challenge the most common misconceptions surrounding BDSM and mental health. It is often believed that individuals who practice BDSM are damaged or mentally ill. In this section, we will examine why this stereotype is harmful and stigmatizing for BDSM practitioners. Additionally, we will cite research that shows no evidence to support the idea that BDSM practitioners are any more likely to have mental health issues than the general population. In fact, we will mention studies that suggest that individuals who practice BDSM may have better mental health outcomes and greater resilience than the general population.

Despite growing acceptance of BDSM in recent years, there remains a widespread belief that individuals who practice BDSM are damaged or mentally ill. This stereotype is not only harmful but also stigmatizing for BDSM practitioners, perpetuating the idea that their desires and practices are deviant or abnormal. However, research has shown that there is no evidence to support the idea that BDSM practitioners are any more likely to have mental health issues than the general population.

A study by Turley (2022) challenges the stereotype of BDSM practitioners as "perverse" or "deviant." The study found that, far from being maladjusted, individuals in the BDSM community are more likely to report greater life satisfaction, positive body image, and social support than those outside the community. Similarly, Hansen-Brown and Jefferson (2022) investigated perceptions of and stigma toward BDSM practitioners, finding that individuals who engaged in BDSM activities did not differ significantly from those who did not engage in BDSM activities in terms of personality traits or psychological characteristics.

Moreover, research has suggested that individuals who practice BDSM may actually have better mental health outcomes and greater resilience than the general population. For instance, a study by Combridge and Lastella (2021) found that individuals with deviant sexual interests, including BDSM practitioners, experienced lower levels of psychological distress and higher levels of self-esteem compared to non-practitioners. This study challenges the commonly held view that individuals who engage in BDSM activities are more likely to be psychologically disturbed than those who do not.

These findings challenge the negative stereotypes that have historically been associated with BDSM, and highlight the need for a more nuanced understanding of this practice. As Turley (2022) notes, BDSM should be understood not as a pathological or deviant behavior but rather as a consensual and healthy form of sexual expression. This is particularly important given the stigmatization that BDSM practitioners face, which can have negative consequences for their mental health and well-being. As research continues to uncover the positive aspects of BDSM, it is important that society begins to view this practice in a more accepting and non-judgmental light.

The Diagnostic and Statistical Manual of Mental Disorders (DSM) has a long and controversial history. The first edition was published in 1952 and has since undergone numerous revisions. The DSM is widely recognized as the authoritative guide to diagnosing mental health conditions in the United States and beyond. However, it has also been subject to criticism and controversy, particularly regarding its inclusion of certain conditions and the process by which those conditions are added or removed. One such condition that was previously included in the DSM was BDSM.

For many years, BDSM was classified as a disorder in the DSM. This classification perpetuated the idea that individuals who practice BDSM are deviant or mentally ill, adding to the stigmatization and marginalization of the BDSM community. It also contributed to a lack of understanding of BDSM and the motivations of those who practice it, leading to further discrimination and prejudice.

It was not until the publication of the DSM-III-R in 1987 that BDSM was officially recognized as a disorder. This classification remained in place until the publication of the DSM-5 in 2013, which removed BDSM from the list of disorders. This change was a significant step forward in the recognition of the legitimacy of BDSM as a healthy and consensual sexual practice. It also challenged the long-standing assumption that individuals who engage in BDSM are mentally ill, paving the way for a more nuanced and evidence-based understanding of BDSM and mental health.

Despite the removal of BDSM as a disorder from the DSM-5, stigma, and discrimination against BDSM practitioners persist. Negative attitudes towards BDSM can lead to social exclusion, discrimination, and even violence against BDSM practitioners. These challenges are further compounded by the lack of legal protections for BDSM practitioners and the difficulties they face in seeking support and treatment from mental health professionals who may lack understanding or knowledge of BDSM.

The stigma against BDSM is not solely based on concerns about mental health, but also reflects broader cultural attitudes about power, gender, and sexuality. The pathologization of BDSM in the DSM and other diagnostic manuals can be traced to historical prejudices and moral judgments against non-normative sexual practices. Despite the increasing acceptance and visibility of BDSM in popular culture, negative attitudes towards BDSM practitioners persist, reflecting deeply ingrained prejudices and misconceptions.

Efforts to challenge stigma against BDSM practitioners must consider broader cultural and political contexts that shape attitudes towards non-normative sexual practices. This includes advocating for legal protections for BDSM practitioners, promoting greater understanding and knowledge of BDSM among mental health professionals, and working to challenge misconceptions and prejudices about BDSM in popular culture. While the removal of BDSM as a disorder from the DSM-5 is an important step in reducing stigma against BDSM, ongoing efforts are needed to promote a more inclusive and accepting approach to sexuality and mental health.

In this section, we have explored the relationship between BDSM and mental health. The commonly held stereotype that individuals who practice BDSM are mentally ill or damaged is not only stigmatizing but also unsupported by research. Studies have shown that those who engage in BDSM may actually have better mental health outcomes and greater resilience than the general population. It is important to view BDSM as a consensual and healthy form of sexual expression, rather than a deviant or pathological behavior. However, stigma and discrimination against BDSM practitioners persist, reflecting broader cultural and political attitudes towards non-normative sexual practices.

The pathologization of BDSM in the Diagnostic and Statistical Manual of Mental Disorders (DSM) contributed to the stigmatization and marginalization of the BDSM community. Despite the removal of BDSM as a disorder from the DSM-5, negative attitudes towards BDSM practitioners persist, and efforts are needed to challenge misconceptions and prejudices about BDSM in popular culture. This includes advocating for legal protections for BDSM practitioners, promoting greater understanding and knowledge of BDSM among mental health professionals, and challenging broader cultural attitudes towards non-normative sexual practices.

It is essential to recognize the importance of safety and consent in BDSM activities, particularly for those who have experienced trauma. BDSM can be both a source of healing and a potential trigger for those with a history of trauma. This highlights the need for a nuanced understanding of the relationship between BDSM and mental health. As research continues to uncover the positive aspects of BDSM, it is vital that society begins to view this practice in a more accepting and non-judgmental light. The removal of BDSM as a disorder from the DSM-5 was a significant step forward in recognizing the legitimacy of BDSM as a consensual and healthy sexual practice. However, ongoing efforts are needed to reduce stigma and promote the well-being of BDSM practitioners.

These negative attitudes towards BDSM practitioners are harmful and stigmatizing, perpetuating the idea that their desires and practices are deviant or abnormal. It is essential to view BDSM as a consensual and healthy form of sexual expression, rather than a pathological or deviant behavior. The pathologization of BDSM in the DSM and other diagnostic manuals can be traced to historical prejudices and moral judgments against non-normative sexual practices. Efforts are needed to challenge stigma and discrimination against BDSM practitioners, including advocating for legal protections, promoting greater understanding among mental health professionals, and working to challenge misconceptions and prejudices about BDSM in popular culture. By doing so, we can create a more accepting and inclusive society for all.

The dangers of engaging in BDSM without proper education and preparation

BDSM is a complex and multifaceted activity that requires a great deal of knowledge, trust, and communication between partners. Engaging in BDSM without proper education and preparation can be a recipe for disaster. The potential risks of BDSM include physical injury, emotional distress, and the violation of consent. It is crucial to approach BDSM with caution and ensure that all parties involved have a clear understanding of what is expected of them, what boundaries are in place, and what measures will be taken to ensure everyone's safety and well-being. In this discussion, we will explore the dangers of engaging in BDSM without proper education and preparation, and the steps that can be taken to mitigate those risks.

It is important to acknowledge the potential dangers of engaging in BDSM without proper education and preparation. The Kink Identity and Sexuality Study (KISS Project) conducted in October 2019 found that individuals who engage in BDSM without proper education and preparation are at a higher risk for experiencing negative physical and psychological effects (Sprott, 2019). This highlights the crucial role that education and preparation play in ensuring the safety and well-being of individuals engaging in BDSM.

Furthermore, the stigma surrounding BDSM can lead to a lack of sex education on the topic, further increasing the risks associated with engaging in it. Another study found that individuals who engage in BDSM may be hesitant to disclose their preferences due to the stigma attached to it. This can lead to a lack of education and preparation, as well as a lack of access to resources that can help ensure safe and consensual BDSM practices.

It is essential to address the stigma and misconceptions surrounding BDSM and promote education and preparation for individuals who choose to engage in it. By doing so, we can help to ensure that those who participate in BDSM do so in a safe, consensual, and informed manner. This will not only reduce the risks associated with BDSM but also promote a more positive and accepting attitude towards individuals who engage in alternative sexual practices.

One way to become more educated and prepared for BDSM activities is to engage in research and reading. This includes reading articles and books on the topic, as well as seeking out credible sources of information online. The Kink Identity and Sexuality Study (KISS Project) conducted by Richard Sprott provides an extensive overview of BDSM practices and identities. This study can be a valuable resource for those who are interested in learning more about the various aspects of BDSM. Additionally, another article on BDSM disclosure and stigma management can be a helpful resource for those who are seeking to navigate the complexities of disclosing their BDSM interests to others.

Another way to become more educated and prepared for BDSM activities is to attend educational workshops and conferences. These events offer a range of opportunities for participants to learn about different aspects of BDSM, including safety practices, negotiation techniques, and communication skills. Many BDSM organizations also offer regular educational programming for their members, providing ongoing opportunities for learning and growth. These workshops and conferences can also be a great way to meet other individuals who share similar interests, providing opportunities for community building and social support.

Based on the potential risks and negative effects associated with engaging in BDSM without proper education and preparation, it is crucial to address the lack of sex education and stigma surrounding BDSM. By promoting education and preparation for individuals who choose to engage in BDSM, we can help ensure safe and consensual practices while reducing the risks associated with this activity. Therefore, this discussion will explore the importance of education and preparation in BDSM, and provide practical ways to mitigate the potential dangers of engaging in BDSM without proper knowledge and preparation.

The risks of physical injuries

When engaging in BDSM activities, there are many potential risks that individuals must be aware of to ensure their safety and well-being. One of the most significant risks is physical injury. BDSM activities often involve physical play, such as spanking, flogging, and bondage, which can result in bruises, cuts, and other injuries. While these injuries are usually minor, they can sometimes be severe or even life-threatening. It is crucial for BDSM practitioners to understand the common types of physical injuries that can occur during BDSM activities, the reasons why they occur, and the safety measures that can be taken to minimize their risk.

Common types of physical injuries that can occur during BDSM activities include bruising, abrasions, cuts, burns, and fractures. These injuries can be caused by a variety of factors, including improper technique, lack of experience, or pushing boundaries too far. While minor injuries such as bruising are relatively common and typically not a cause for concern, more severe injuries such as fractures and burns can result in permanent damage and even disability. It is important to note that the risk of physical injury can vary depending on the type of activity and the level of experience of the participants involved. Therefore, it is crucial for individuals engaging in BDSM activities to have a thorough understanding of the risks associated with each activity and to take appropriate safety measures.

BDSM activities can pose a significant risk of physical injury to participants. Severe acute kidney injury is one such risk that has been reported in medical literature. A case report published in **BMJ Case Reports** described a man who developed acute kidney injury after engaging in violent sadomasochistic play (Echterdiek et al., 2018). The play involved the use of a device designed to restrict blood flow to the penis. As a result of the injury, the man required haemodialysis and was at risk of long-term kidney damage.

Other injuries commonly associated with BDSM activities include bruises, burns, cuts, and abrasions. A literature review conducted by Schori et al. (2021) found that while fatal outcomes in BDSM play are rare, they do occur. The authors analyzed 33 cases of fatal outcomes related to BDSM play and found that the most common cause of death was asphyxia. Other causes of death included trauma, intoxication, and medical conditions exacerbated by BDSM play.

Some common injuries that can occur during BDSM activities include:

- Bruises
- Burns
- Cuts
- Abrasions
- Acute kidney injury
- Asphyxia
- Trauma
- Intoxication
- Medical conditions exacerbated by BDSM play

While not all BDSM activities are inherently dangerous, the risks of physical injury should not be ignored. It is crucial for individuals engaging in BDSM to be aware of these risks and to take appropriate measures to mitigate them. This may include utilizing safety equipment, such as restraints, paddles, or whips designed for BDSM play, and ensuring that all participants have a clear understanding of what activities will take place and what limits are in place. Furthermore, it is essential for individuals engaging in BDSM to have a thorough understanding of anatomy and physiology, particularly when engaging in activities that involve pressure or constriction. By taking these precautions, individuals can help ensure that they engage in BDSM activities in a responsible and safe manner.

Engaging in BDSM activities without proper safety measures and knowledge of anatomy can lead to various physical injuries. The nature of BDSM activities, which often include physically intense acts such as bondage, impact play, and suspension, can result in strains, sprains, bruises, bone fractures, and organ damage. Practitioners may also engage in activities that involve choking or cutting, which can cause serious injuries or even death.

Another factor that contributes to injuries in BDSM is the lack of communication and trust between partners. BDSM activities require a high level of trust and communication to ensure that both parties are comfortable and safe and that boundaries are respected. When partners fail to communicate clearly, they may engage in activities that go beyond their limits and lead to physical harm. In some cases, partners may ignore or violate each other's boundaries, resulting in serious physical harm.

A lack of education and preparation is also a common cause of injuries in BDSM activities. Due to the stigma surrounding BDSM, it can be difficult for practitioners to access information and resources on how to practice BDSM safely. This lack of education can lead to improper use of BDSM equipment or failure to recognize the signs of injury, resulting in more severe harm.

In the world of BDSM, safety measures and knowledge about anatomy play a crucial role in ensuring that practitioners can engage in activities without causing harm to themselves or their partners. Wuyts and Morrens (2022) conducted a systematic review of the biology of BDSM and found that practitioners who were well-versed in anatomy were better equipped to prevent injuries during physically intense activities such as impact play and suspension. The study also highlighted the importance of proper use of BDSM equipment, which can reduce the risk of injury during bondage or other activities.

Wuyts et al. (2020) conducted a pilot study on the biological mechanisms associated with BDSM interactions in dominants and submissives. The study found that participants who had a good understanding of anatomy and were able to communicate their boundaries clearly experienced more positive outcomes during BDSM activities. The study emphasizes the importance of communication and trust between partners, as well as the need for practitioners to have a basic understanding of anatomy and the potential risks associated with certain activities.

Furthermore, Wuyts et al. (2020) noted that the stigma surrounding BDSM can make it difficult for practitioners to access information and resources on how to practice BDSM safely. The lack of education and preparation can contribute to injuries in BDSM activities and increase the risk of severe harm. It is crucial for practitioners to seek out educational resources and to communicate openly with their partners about their boundaries and preferences to ensure a safe and enjoyable experience for all parties involved.

The risks of psychological harm

While BDSM can be a safe and enjoyable way for consenting adults to explore their sexuality and emotions, it is not without its risks. One of the potential risks of BDSM is psychological harm, which can result from a variety of factors, including the intense emotions that can arise during BDSM activities, the power dynamics inherent in BDSM relationships, and the potential for non-consensual activities or violations of boundaries. In this section, we will explore the impact of BDSM activities on mental health, the role of communication and consent in preventing psychological harm, and the importance of understanding power dynamics and aftercare in maintaining healthy BDSM relationships.

Chapter 1 introduced us to the concept of BDSM and its impact on mental health. That chapter explored the various factors that contribute to the psychological effects of BDSM activities, including the individual's personal experiences, past traumas, and the nature of the activities themselves. It also emphasizes the importance of understanding the complex relationship between BDSM and mental health to promote a safe and responsible practice of BDSM.

In addition to these points, it is important to note that Chapter 1 also discusses the potential risks and benefits of BDSM activities on mental health. Some practitioners report positive experiences and psychological benefits such as increased intimacy and emotional connection with their partners. However, it also highlights the potential negative impact of BDSM on mental health, particularly when it is not practiced safely, consensually, and responsibly.

There is a need for a nuanced and informed approach to the impact of BDSM on mental health. Focusing on the importance of open communication, consent, and understanding of one's own limits and boundaries to prevent psychological harm.

Effective communication and informed consent are essential in preventing psychological harm in BDSM activities (Brown et al. 2019). BDSM practitioners should have open and honest communication about their expectations, boundaries, and limitations before engaging in any activities (Ten Brink et al., 2020). Consent should be explicit, ongoing, and informed, meaning that all parties involved fully understand the risks and benefits of the activities and are freely consenting to them (Brown et al., 2019). Practitioners should also be aware of the power dynamics at play in BDSM activities and ensure that they are not exploiting or coercing their partners (Ten Brink et al., 2020).

Research has shown that communication and consent are important in reducing the risk of psychological harm in BDSM activities (Brown et al., 2019; Ten Brink et al., 2020). However, practitioners may face barriers to effective communication, such as shame, embarrassment, or fear of rejection (Brown et al., 2019). It is important for practitioners to understand that open communication is not only necessary but also beneficial for the well-being of all parties involved (Ten Brink et al., 2020). They should also prioritize consent to establish mutual respect and trust between partners.

Furthermore, practitioners should be aware of the potential risks associated with certain BDSM activities and communicate these risks to their partners (Brown et al., 2019). For example, activities that involve physical restraint, impact play, or breath play can pose a risk of physical harm if not executed properly. Practitioners should educate themselves on proper technique and safety measures and have a plan in place for emergencies (Ten Brink et al., 2020). Consensual non-consent, or play that involves a negotiated lack of consent, can also pose a risk of psychological harm, and should be approached with caution (Brown et al., 2019).

The importance of understanding power dynamics and aftercare

The importance of understanding power dynamics in BDSM cannot be overstated. Cutler et al. (2020) investigated how self-defined long-term BDSM couples selected their partners and navigated power dynamics within their relationships. Their research revealed that power dynamics were highly individualized and were often negotiated and renegotiated throughout the course of the relationship. Communication played a crucial role in establishing and maintaining the power dynamics within these relationships.

Simula (2019) reviewed the literature on the experiences of BDSM participants and found that power dynamics were central to the BDSM experience. Participants found that power exchange was a way to explore their own limits and push beyond them. They also found that power exchange was a way to create intimacy and trust within their relationships. However, power exchange also presented unique challenges, such as the potential for emotional and psychological harm.

In a qualitative study of dominant and submissive BDSM roles, Hébert and Weaver (2015) found that power dynamics were often enacted through role-playing and negotiation. Dominants found pleasure in being able to control their partner's experience, while submissives found pleasure in surrendering control. The authors note that these dynamics can be used to create positive experiences for both partners, but caution that power exchange can also be abused.

Understanding power dynamics in BDSM requires communication, negotiation, and ongoing consent. Participants must have a deep understanding of their own limits and boundaries, and be able to articulate them to their partners. Additionally, participants must be able to read their partner's cues and respond to them appropriately. The power dynamics within BDSM relationships are highly individualized and must be negotiated and renegotiated over time to ensure that both partners feel safe and supported.

Understanding and respecting power dynamics is crucial in preventing harm and promoting a safe and consensual BDSM experience. However, it is not the only aspect that practitioners should consider. Aftercare, which refers to the emotional and physical care given to participants after a BDSM scene or session, is another important component of responsible BDSM practices. In the next section, we will discuss the significance of aftercare and how it can help mitigate potential psychological harm.

Aftercare is an essential aspect of BDSM, which often involves physical and psychological intensity. The dominant and submissive roles can be emotionally charged and, as such, require aftercare to promote the physical and emotional safety of all parties involved. According to

Fuentes (2019), aftercare is crucial to mitigating potential negative outcomes of BDSM activities. A lack of aftercare can lead to feelings of isolation, guilt, and shame, among other adverse psychological effects.

Gunning et al. (2023) explored the intersections of sexual communication in BDSM and disability, emphasizing the need for disability-inclusive aftercare. The study found that participants with disabilities perceived aftercare to counteract the potential harm associated with BDSM activities. This highlights the need for BDSM practitioners to consider the needs of all parties involved, including individuals with disabilities, and prioritize their safety and wellbeing. By doing so, it ensures that BDSM practices are inclusive and accessible to everyone.

Additionally, the provision of aftercare can lead to positive emotional experiences that enhance relationships and facilitate personal growth. Fuentes (2019) found that aftercare fosters feelings of trust and emotional closeness between partners, and contributes to long-term relationship satisfaction. Thus, aftercare can strengthen the bonds between partners and reinforce the positive aspects of BDSM practices, ultimately leading to a healthier and more fulfilling sexual life.

The importance of aftercare cannot be overstated in the BDSM community. It is necessary to ensure the physical and emotional safety of all parties involved, promote relationship satisfaction, and facilitate personal growth. By prioritizing aftercare, practitioners can create a positive and inclusive environment that promotes safety, trust, and emotional closeness.

BDSM can be a highly rewarding practice for those who engage in it, but it also comes with inherent risks of physical and psychological harm. It is crucial to prioritize education and preparation to minimize these risks and ensure the safety of all participants. This includes understanding the importance of communication and consent, as well as recognizing and navigating power dynamics within BDSM relationships. Moreover, providing aftercare for all parties involved is essential to facilitate emotional healing and promote the overall well-being of everyone involved.

As we move forward, it is vital for BDSM practitioners to acknowledge these risks and prioritize responsible and safe practices. By educating ourselves and taking necessary precautions, we can create a more inclusive and empowering environment for all those involved. Ultimately, it is up to each of us to do our part in ensuring that BDSM remains a safe and consensual practice that promotes emotional and physical well-being.

BDSM is an activity that requires a great deal of education and preparation to be done responsibly and safely. With the potential risks of physical and psychological harm, it is essential that BDSM practitioners prioritize their education and preparation before engaging in any activities. The lack of proper education and preparation can lead to severe and lasting harm to oneself and one's partner. Therefore, it is imperative that BDSM practitioners take the time to learn about the various aspects of BDSM, including the risks and the proper use of equipment, before engaging in any activities.

One way for BDSM practitioners to prioritize their education and preparation is by attending workshops or training sessions on BDSM. These sessions provide a safe and supportive environment for individuals to learn about BDSM and develop their skills. Additionally, BDSM practitioners can seek out experienced mentors who can guide them through the learning process and offer advice and support. By prioritizing education and preparation, BDSM practitioners can reduce the risks associated with BDSM and ensure that their activities are conducted safely and responsibly.

Responsible and safe BDSM practices are critical to ensure the well-being of all participants involved. As we have discussed, there are inherent risks of physical and psychological harm in BDSM activities that cannot be ignored. Therefore, education and preparation are essential for BDSM practitioners to engage in these activities safely and responsibly.

Furthermore, it is essential to acknowledge the importance of power dynamics and aftercare in BDSM practices. Dominant-submissive relationships and power exchange can be consensual, but it is crucial to ensure that these dynamics do not lead to harm or abuse. Proper aftercare ensures that participants receive the necessary emotional and physical support after engaging in BDSM activities.

BDSM activities are a valid and consensual way for adults to explore their sexuality and desires. However, the importance of safety and responsibility cannot be overstated. Practitioners must prioritize education, preparation, and aftercare to ensure that they engage in these activities safely and responsibly. Only then can BDSM activities be a healthy and fulfilling part of adult sexuality.

Navigating the stigma around BDSM and mental health

BDSM practitioners face negative perceptions and discrimination because of their sexual preferences and practices. Society often views BDSM as deviant behavior and as a result, many practitioners are stigmatized and marginalized. This stigma can lead to a lack of social support and negative mental health outcomes, such as anxiety and depression. Hansen-Brown and Jefferson (2022) found that discrimination towards BDSM practitioners can be due to misconceptions, lack of knowledge, and moral judgments of those who are not familiar with the BDSM culture.

Negative media perceptions also contribute to the stigma surrounding BDSM. In movies and television shows, BDSM is often portrayed as abusive or deviant, further fueling the public's negative perceptions. These depictions can reinforce stereotypes and contribute to the discrimination of BDSM practitioners. It is important for media outlets to portray BDSM in an accurate and non-judgmental way to help reduce the stigma surrounding it.

Despite the negative perceptions, BDSM practitioners can overcome the challenges they face by advocating for their community and educating the public about BDSM. Practitioners can work towards breaking down stereotypes and increasing awareness about the BDSM culture. They can also provide education to those who may not be familiar with the practices and work towards dispelling misconceptions.

BDSM practitioners can also create and seek out safe spaces where they can feel supported and understood. These spaces can provide a sense of community and help reduce feelings of isolation and discrimination. They can also provide opportunities for practitioners to educate others about the BDSM culture and its practices.

It is also important for BDSM practitioners to prioritize their mental health and seek out mental health professionals who are knowledgeable about BDSM practices. Mental health professionals who are unfamiliar with BDSM may pathologize it or view it as a disorder, which can be harmful to their clients. Seeking out professionals who are knowledgeable about BDSM can lead to more positive mental health outcomes for practitioners.

Navigating the stigma surrounding BDSM and mental health can be challenging for practitioners. Negative perceptions and discrimination can lead to feelings of shame, guilt, and secrecy, and can deter individuals from seeking help when needed. Negative media portrayals and entertainment perceptions in movies and television can also contribute to negative attitudes and stereotypes about BDSM. Despite these challenges, practitioners can take steps to overcome these obstacles, such as seeking out supportive communities and engaging in open communication with partners and healthcare providers. By promoting education, understanding, and acceptance of BDSM, practitioners can work towards reducing stigma and improving access to care for individuals who engage in this practice.

Chapter 6

The Intersection of Psychology and BDSM

We understand that BDSM is a complex and multitiered practice that has gained increased attention in last few decades. While some may view BDSM solely as a form of sexual expression, it also encompasses emotional and psychological components that contribute to the overall experience. In this chapter, we will explore the intersection of psychology and BDSM, and how the two can inform and enrich each other.

The field of psychology has much to offer in terms of understanding the motivations and experiences of individuals engaged in BDSM. By examining BDSM through a psychological lens, we can gain insight into how individuals engage in the practice, what they hope to gain from it, and how it affects their overall well-being. At the same time, BDSM can also shed light on various psychological theories and concepts, such as power dynamics, attachment styles, and trauma.

Moreover, the intersection of psychology and BDSM is not limited to individual experiences. As a social phenomenon, BDSM also involves group dynamics and cultural factors. Understanding the psychological underpinnings of BDSM can help us understand the norms, values, and practices of BDSM communities and how they shape the experiences of their members. In this chapter, we will explore these different dimensions of the intersection of psychology and BDSM, and how they can inform our understanding of this complex and fascinating practice.

The role of psychology in BDSM experiences

BDSM has been the subject of considerable study in recent years. A key focus of this research has been the psychological characteristics of BDSM practitioners. Wismeijer and van Assen (2013) found that BDSM practitioners had higher levels of extraversion, openness to experience, and conscientiousness compared to non-practitioners. This suggests that people who engage in BDSM may be more willing to take risks, be more creative, and have a greater sense of responsibility. However, the study also found that BDSM practitioners reported lower levels of neuroticism compared to non-practitioners, indicating that they may be less anxious and more emotionally stable.

Despite growing acceptance of BDSM in mainstream society, there is still a stigma surrounding the practice. A study by Schuerwegen et al. (2022) investigated the role of stigma and psychological mechanisms in BDSM experiences. The study found that BDSM practitioners experienced higher levels of internalized stigma compared to non-practitioners, which may have negative effects on their mental health and well-being. However, the study also found that BDSM practitioners reported higher levels of self-esteem and subjective well-being compared to non-practitioners, suggesting that engaging in BDSM may have positive psychological effects.

Research has also explored the relationship between BDSM interests and trauma and attachment styles. Ten Brink et al. (2020) found that individuals with a history of childhood trauma were more likely to report an interest in BDSM. The study also found that individuals with a secure attachment style reported less interest in BDSM, while those with an anxious or avoidant attachment style reported more interest. This suggests that early attachment experiences may play a role in the development of BDSM interests.

Qualitative research has also been conducted to explore the experiences of individuals in dominant and submissive roles in BDSM. Hébert and Weaver (2015) conducted a study that explored the perks and problems associated with these roles. The study found that individuals in dominant roles experienced benefits such as increased self-confidence and a sense of control, while individuals in submissive roles experienced benefits such as stress relief and increased intimacy with their partner. However, the study also found that both dominant and submissive individuals faced challenges such as finding compatible partners and dealing with societal stigma.

One hypothesis that has been proposed to explain the appeal of BDSM is an evolutionary one. Dahan (2019) suggests that BDSM practices may have evolved as a way for humans to cope with stress and pain. The author proposes that sexual masochism may have evolved to release endorphins and reduce stress, while sexual sadism may have evolved as a way to assert dominance and reduce competition for resources. This hypothesis highlights the potential adaptive functions of BDSM practices and underscores the importance of understanding them from an evolutionary perspective.

Overall, the role of psychology in BDSM experiences is a complex and multifaceted one. Research has shed light on the psychological characteristics of BDSM practitioners, the effects of stigma and psychological mechanisms on their experiences, the relationship between trauma and attachment styles and BDSM interests, and the perks and problems associated with dominant and submissive roles. Further research is needed to deepen our understanding of the psychological aspects of BDSM and to help reduce the stigma surrounding this practice.

How to approach BDSM through a psychological lens

BDSM has been a topic of interest for psychologists due to its unconventional and potentially stigmatized nature. To approach BDSM through a psychological lens, one must consider the prevalence, etiological, psychological, and interpersonal factors associated with BDSM, as outlined in a systematic scoping review by Brown et al. (2019). The review highlights that BDSM is not uncommon, and the factors associated with it are complex and multifaceted. Understanding the various factors can help to increase acceptance and reduce stigma surrounding the practice.

In addition to prevalence and etiological factors, understanding the psychological motivations behind BDSM is crucial. Turley et al. (2018) conducted a study on the erotic experiences of BDSM practitioners, emphasizing the importance of pleasure and the desire for intensity and novelty. For some, BDSM can provide a sense of escape from everyday life, while for others, it can be a form of self-exploration. Pietrusza (2019) provides a theoretical framework for BDSM, discussing the importance of personal agency and self-acceptance in BDSM practices.

While BDSM can be a fulfilling and consensual activity, it is not without risks. BDSM practitioners need to ensure that their activities are safe, sane, and consensual. Simula (2019) reviews the literature on the experiences of BDSM participants, highlighting the need for communication, trust, and negotiation between partners. Establishing boundaries and respecting them is essential to the safety and well-being of all parties involved.

Moreover, it is important to recognize that BDSM practices can have implications for interpersonal relationships. BDSM activities can help to establish intimacy and trust between partners, but they can also lead to power imbalances and the reinforcement of gender stereotypes. Simula's (2021) special issue on BDSM studies emphasizes the need for a nuanced understanding of the complexities of BDSM practices, recognizing that they are influenced by broader cultural and societal norms.

One potential psychological framework that can be used to understand BDSM is attachment theory. Attachment theory suggests that individuals develop specific attachment styles based on their early experiences with caregivers, and these attachment styles influence their subsequent relationships and behaviors (Mikulincer & Shaver, 2016). For example, individuals with a secure attachment style tend to have positive self-esteem, trust others, and have satisfying interpersonal relationships. In the context of BDSM, individuals with a secure attachment style may be more likely to engage in consensual and mutually satisfying BDSM practices. On the other hand, individuals with an anxious attachment style may have a heightened need for validation and reassurance from their partners, which could manifest in seeking out BDSM experiences that provide a sense of control or validation. Individuals with an avoidant attachment style, who tend to avoid intimacy and emotional vulnerability, may be drawn to BDSM to engage in sexual experiences without emotional intimacy. Understanding how attachment styles relate to BDSM practices can provide important insights into how individuals navigate their desires and relationships in the BDSM community.

Finally, it is important to acknowledge that BDSM is not necessarily pathological or deviant behavior. Williams et al. (2016) conducted a study on the recreational nature of BDSM, finding that the participants experienced psychological well-being and enhanced intimacy with their partners. Recognizing the normality of BDSM can help to reduce the stigma and discrimination experienced by practitioners.

Ultimately, approaching BDSM through a psychological lens requires an understanding of the various factors associated with it, the psychological motivations behind it, the importance of safety and communication, the implications for interpersonal relationships, and the normality of BDSM. Understanding these factors can increase acceptance and reduce stigma surrounding BDSM practices, focused on promoting the well-being and safety of practitioners.

Chapter 7

Cultivating Healthy BDSM Practices

Cultivating healthy BDSM practices is a critical aspect of engaging in BDSM that ensures physical and psychological safety, pleasure, and personal growth. A healthy BDSM practice begins with establishing boundaries, developing communication skills, and fostering mutual respect between partners. These elements enable partners to engage in BDSM activities that are consensual and safe, while also allowing them to express their desires and explore their sexuality. Developing healthy BDSM practices requires time, patience, and dedication, but the benefits are significant, leading to improved relationships, self-awareness, and overall well-being.

One strategy for cultivating healthy BDSM practices is the development of a safe word. A safe word is a mutually agreed-upon term that partners use during BDSM activities to communicate that they want to stop or slow down the activities. The use of a safe word can prevent harm to either partner and can serve as a useful tool in building trust and respect. In addition, practicing active listening and empathy can promote healthy communication and increase intimacy in BDSM relationships. Partners who actively listen to each other and demonstrate empathy during BDSM activities are better able to understand each other's needs and desires and can create an environment where both partners feel safe and comfortable.

Building a positive BDSM community is another critical strategy for cultivating healthy BDSM practices. A positive BDSM community provides a supportive and non-judgmental environment that fosters growth, education, and empowerment. Communities that promote positive BDSM practices encourage communication, education, and safe exploration. In addition, a positive BDSM community provides resources and support for individuals who may be struggling with BDSM-related issues, including shame, guilt, or anxiety. Individuals who are part of a positive BDSM community can experience increased self-esteem, self-awareness, and a sense of belonging.

Balancing BDSM with other aspects of life is essential for cultivating a healthy BDSM practice. Balancing BDSM with other aspects of life involves setting boundaries and prioritizing self-care. For example, individuals who engage in BDSM should ensure that they are getting enough rest, eating well, and engaging in other self-care practices. Moreover, partners should balance BDSM activities with other activities that promote well-being, such as hobbies, socializing with friends and family, and exercise. Balancing BDSM with other aspects of life can help individuals maintain a healthy balance and avoid burnout or other negative consequences.

Cultivating healthy BDSM practices involves developing strategies that promote clear communication, self-care, building a positive community, and balancing BDSM with other life aspects. By prioritizing healthy practices, individuals can engage in BDSM activities in a safe, consensual, and positive manner.

Strategies for fostering a healthy BDSM practice

Cultivating a healthy BDSM practice involves implementing strategies that promote a safe, consensual, and positive experience for all participants. BDSM activities involve power dynamics, and it is essential to develop effective strategies that prioritize the well-being of all parties involved. These strategies can include communication, boundary-setting, and self-care practices. By prioritizing healthy practices, individuals can engage in BDSM activities in a way that promotes mutual respect, trust, and intimacy.

One strategy for fostering a healthy BDSM practice is through clear communication. Communication is essential for establishing and maintaining boundaries, expressing desires and needs, and ensuring that all parties involved are comfortable and consenting to the activity. Effective communication can be facilitated by safewords, which provide a way for participants to communicate when they want to stop the activity. In addition, open communication can enable partners to discuss their experiences, preferences, and limits to ensure that they are on the same wavelength.

Another strategy for fostering a healthy BDSM practice is to prioritize self-care. BDSM activities can be physically and emotionally demanding, and it is important to engage in self-care practices to promote well-being. This can include taking breaks when needed, engaging in relaxing activities, and seeking support when necessary. Self-care is especially important for individuals who have experienced past trauma, as BDSM activities may trigger traumatic experiences.

Overall, strategies for fostering a healthy BDSM practice involve prioritizing effective communication, establishing, and maintaining boundaries, and engaging in self-care practices. By implementing these strategies, individuals can create a safe and positive environment for engaging in BDSM activities.

There are various strategies that can foster a healthy BDSM practice. From communication to self-reflection, these strategies can help individuals navigate the complexities of BDSM and ensure a safe and consensual experience. Below are five ways to promote healthy BDSM practices.

- Develop a clear and comprehensive BDSM contract
- Practice active listening and effective communication
- Engage in self-reflection and self-care
- Set and respect boundaries and limits
- Continuously educate oneself and stay informed about safe BDSM practices

Develop a clear and comprehensive BDSM contract: A BDSM contract can help partners establish their roles, boundaries, and expectations. This contract can include a detailed description of activities that will be engaged in, as well as any limits or restrictions. It is important to review and update the contract regularly to ensure that it is still relevant and reflective of the participants' desires and needs.

Practice active listening and effective communication: Communication is key in any healthy BDSM practice. Active listening involves paying attention to one's partner, asking questions, and clarifying any misunderstandings. Effective communication involves expressing one's desires, boundaries, and needs, as well as being receptive to one's partner's feedback.

Engage in self-reflection and self-care: BDSM activities can be physically and emotionally demanding. Engaging in self-reflection and self-care can help participants navigate these demands and promote overall well-being. This can include taking breaks when needed, engaging in relaxing activities, and seeking support when necessary.

Set and respect boundaries and limits: Boundaries and limits are essential components of any healthy BDSM practice. Partners should discuss and agree on their boundaries and limits before engaging in any activities. It is important to respect each other's boundaries and to communicate any changes or updates.

Continuously educate oneself and stay informed about safe BDSM practices: BDSM practices and safety guidelines are constantly evolving. It is important to stay informed about any changes and updates in order to engage in safe and consensual BDSM activities. This can include reading books, attending workshops, or seeking advice from experienced BDSM practitioners.

Fostering a healthy BDSM practice is essential for individuals to ensure they engage in BDSM activities in a safe and consensual manner. Through communication, participants can clearly express their desires and limits with their partner(s). Practicing self-care is another important strategy to prevent emotional and physical burnout during BDSM activities. Building a positive BDSM community can provide support and help participants learn safe and consensual practices. Balancing BDSM activities with other areas of life can help prevent individuals from becoming consumed by BDSM and ensure they can engage in other aspects of their lives without feeling overwhelmed. Finally, being aware of one's strengths and using them in BDSM activities can lead to a more positive experience. By incorporating these strategies into their BDSM practices, individuals can prioritize their physical, emotional, and psychological well-being while engaging in consensual BDSM activities.

Tips for building a positive BDSM community

Building a positive BDSM community is essential for those who practice BDSM as it provides a sense of belonging, support, and education. Communities are a space where people can share experiences, learn new skills, and connect with like-minded individuals. However, creating and sustaining a community that is inclusive, safe, and supportive requires intentionality, effort, and a shared commitment to respect, communication, effort, and consent.

In this section, we will explore some different ways that can help individuals build a positive BDSM community. These tips are not exhaustive but offer a starting point for anyone looking to create and sustain a healthy community. By following these tips, individuals can create a space that is welcoming and supportive, where members feel free to explore their desires and share their experiences.

Here are the five tips for building a positive BDSM community:

- Foster a culture of consent

- Create opportunities for education and learning
- Encourage open and respectful communication
- Promote diversity and inclusivity
- Organize safe and inclusive events

Let us delve into each of these tips in more detail:

1. Foster a culture of consent: Consent is the cornerstone of BDSM practices, and it should also guide the formation and maintenance of BDSM communities. Creating a culture of consent means prioritizing the needs and boundaries of individuals, providing education on consent, and empowering members to advocate for their own needs and boundaries.

2. Create opportunities for education and learning: Education is crucial in promoting safe and consensual BDSM practices. Communities can offer educational resources, workshops, and training sessions that cover a range of topics, from safety protocols to negotiation skills.

3. Encourage open and respectful communication: Effective communication is essential in BDSM practices and in building healthy communities. Encouraging open and respectful communication means creating spaces where members feel comfortable expressing their needs and concerns, active listening, and resolving conflicts in a constructive manner.

4. Promote diversity and inclusivity: BDSM communities should aim to be diverse and inclusive, welcoming individuals of all genders, sexual orientations, races, and abilities. Promoting diversity and inclusivity means actively seeking out and welcoming individuals from underrepresented communities, challenging discrimination, prejudice, and creating a culture of respect and support.

5. Organize safe and inclusive events: Events are an essential part of BDSM communities, and organizers have a responsibility to create events that are safe and inclusive for all members. This means establishing clear safety protocols, providing education and resources, and actively addressing and preventing harassment and discrimination.

Creating and sustaining a positive BDSM community is essential to the well-being of individuals who participate in BDSM practices. By following the five tips outlined above, communities can foster an environment of safety, inclusivity, and respect. It is important to keep in mind that building a positive BDSM community is an ongoing process that requires effort, intentionality, and a willingness to learn from mistakes. It is essential to recognize that everyone in the community has a role to play in creating and maintaining a supportive environment, and to promote a culture of consent, respect, and communication.

As BDSM continues to gain wider acceptance, communities have an important role to play in promoting education, challenging stigma, and providing a space for individuals to connect and explore their interests. By working together to build positive BDSM communities, we can create a safer, more inclusive, and more fulfilling space for everyone involved.

Balancing BDSM with other aspects of life

Balancing BDSM with other aspects of life can be challenging for individuals who enjoy engaging in BDSM practices. BDSM can be time-consuming, emotionally draining, and physically demanding, which can make it difficult to maintain a healthy balance with work, family, and other obligations. It is important to ensure that BDSM practices do not interfere with other areas of life, and that one is able to enjoy BDSM in a way that is safe, responsible, and sustainable.

Achieving balance requires intentional effort and a commitment to self-care. It is important to prioritize self-care practices to ensure physical, mental, and emotional well-being. Setting boundaries and communicating them clearly is also essential for maintaining a healthy balance. Creating a schedule and sticking to it can help in ensuring that BDSM practices do not interfere with other obligations. Involving partners and loved ones in BDSM practices can promote a sense of understanding and support for one's lifestyle. Seeking support from like-minded individuals can provide a sense of community and help with maintaining a healthy balance.

We will explore five tips for balancing BDSM with other aspects of life. These tips are in no way exhaustive and may provide some guidance on how to enjoy BDSM practices in a way that is sustainable and fulfilling, while also ensuring that other areas of life are not neglected. Five tips for balancing BDSM with other aspects of life:

- Prioritize self-care
- Set boundaries and communicate them clearly
- Create a schedule and stick to it
- Involve partners and loved ones in BDSM practices
- Seek support from like-minded individuals

Let us delve into each of these tips in more detail:

1. Prioritizing self-care means taking care of one's physical, emotional, and mental health. This can include activities such as exercise, meditation, therapy, or simply taking time for oneself to relax and recharge.

2. Setting boundaries is important in any relationship, but especially in BDSM practices where the lines between play and reality can become blurred. Communicating those boundaries clearly and consistently can prevent misunderstandings and promote trust and respect.

3. Creating a schedule for BDSM activities and sticking to it can help individuals balance their BDSM practices with other responsibilities and obligations. It can also provide a sense of structure and predictability, which can reduce stress and anxiety.

4. Involving partners and loved ones in BDSM practices can help individuals maintain a healthy balance between their BDSM lifestyle and their other relationships. This can involve discussing boundaries and expectations, finding ways to include partners in BDSM activities, or simply being open and honest about one's interests and desires.

5. Seeking support from like-minded individuals can provide a sense of community and belonging. This can involve joining a BDSM group or attending events, finding a mentor or teacher, or simply connecting with others online.

Balancing BDSM with other aspects of life requires a thoughtful and intentional approach to ensure a healthy and fulfilling practice. By prioritizing self-care, setting clear boundaries, creating a manageable schedule, involving loved ones, and seeking support, individuals can navigate the demands of their daily lives while maintaining their BDSM practice. It's essential to remember that everyone's journey is unique, and it may take some time and experimentation to find the right balance. However, by following these tips and making self-care a priority, individuals can create a sustainable and fulfilling BDSM practice that complements the other aspects of their lives.

Chapter 8

Bringing it All Together

This book is a culmination of BDSM experiences and psychology and seeks to connect the dots between the different topics and themes explored in the preceding chapters. At its core, emphasizing the importance of understanding BDSM as a holistic practice that encompasses physical, emotional, and psychological components. This has allowed the exploration of the intersection between BDSM and Psychology. It expanded on the introduction to BDSM, as a term that encompasses a range of sexual practices involving consensual power exchange between partners. Although the BDSM lifestyle has become more visible in recent years, there is still a lack of understanding and education around BDSM, particularly in its connection to mental health. This provided the opportunity to address this gap by exploring the psychological impacts of BDSM and the importance of cultivating healthy BDSM practices.

In healthy BDSM relationships, all parties involved understand and have consented to the activities taking place. Communication at its core, is essential to ensure that all parties understand each other's boundaries and that these boundaries are respected. This is especially important when considering the potential impact of trauma on BDSM activities. Childhood trauma, such as physical, emotional, or sexual abuse, can have a profound impact on an individual's psychological development and can shape their relationship with power and control in adulthood. Individuals who have experienced childhood trauma may be more likely to engage in BDSM activities as a way of processing and coping with past experiences of abuse.

We explored one of the psychological responses that can accompany BDSM. Dissociation is an altered state of consciousness that can be both positive and negative, but it is important to understand how it impacts individuals who engage in BDSM play. This allowed a deeper exploration into the psychology behind dissociation in BDSM, the potential impacts it can have, and coping mechanisms that can be used to minimize negative experiences.

We looked at the misconceptions and stigma surrounding BDSM and its practitioners. Despite its growing popularity and acceptance, many people still hold misconceptions about what BDSM is, and how it relates to mental health. The book explores some of the most common pitfalls and misconceptions surrounding BDSM, and how they can impact mental health.

The intersection of psychology and BDSM allowed the examination components within. While some may view BDSM solely as a form of sexual expression, it also encompasses emotional and psychological components that contribute to the overall experience. It allowed the connection of how the two can inform and enrich each other, highlighting the potential benefits of engaging in BDSM activities, such as improved relationships, self-awareness, and overall well-being.

Finally, looking at the importance of cultivating healthy BDSM practices. This includes establishing boundaries, developing communication skills, and fostering mutual respect between partners and the BDSM community. By doing so, partners can engage in BDSM activities that are consensual and safe, while also allowing them to express their desires and explore their sexuality. Developing healthy BDSM practices requires time, patience, and dedication, but the benefits are significant. It allowed us to develop bonds with people from all walks of life there for the love of BDSM.

Overall, this was an attempt at a comprehensive exploration of the psychological impacts of BDSM and the importance of cultivating healthy BDSM practices. By doing so, individuals and partners can engage in BDSM activities in a safe and consensual manner, leading to improved relationships, self-awareness, and overall well-being.

Reflecting on the importance of healthy BDSM practices for mental health

From a philosophical standpoint, healthy BDSM practices can be viewed as a means of exploring and expressing the human condition. BDSM allows individuals to explore the various facets of power exchange and control, which are inherent to human relationships. By engaging in these practices in a safe and consensual manner, individuals can explore their desires and boundaries, develop self-awareness, and cultivate a sense of agency and control over their lives.

BDSM practices can also serve as a coping mechanism, particularly for individuals who have experienced trauma or abuse. By engaging in consensual power exchange, individuals can reframe their experiences of powerlessness and reclaim control over their lives. This process can be empowering and transformative, leading to improved mental health outcomes.

Moreover, healthy BDSM practices can foster a sense of community and belonging, particularly for those who may feel marginalized or misunderstood in mainstream society. By providing a safe and judgment-free space for individuals to express their desires and identities, healthy BDSM practices can promote self-acceptance and validation. This sense of belonging and community can lead to greater social connectedness and improved mental health outcomes. Philosophically, BDSM practices can be viewed as a celebration of human diversity and complexity, and a means of promoting individual and collective well-being, something we all should strive for.

Encouragement to continue exploring the connection between BDSM and mental health

As we come to the end of this book, it is important to recognize that our exploration of the connection between BDSM and mental health is far from complete. While we have examined many aspects of healthy BDSM practices and their potential benefits for mental health, there is still much to be explored and understood.

One area where further research is needed is in understanding the psychological processes involved in BDSM. Despite the growing acceptance and visibility of BDSM in mainstream culture, there is still a significant lack of understanding about the motivations and experiences of those who engage in these practices. By conducting research on the psychological processes involved in BDSM, we can gain a better understanding of the potential benefits and risks associated with these practices, and develop more effective interventions and support services for those who engage in them.

Another area where further exploration is needed is in understanding the diversity of experiences within the BDSM community. While we have focused primarily on the potential benefits of healthy BDSM practices, it is important to recognize that not all BDSM experiences are positive or healthy. There are many factors that can contribute to negative experiences, including trauma, abuse, and discrimination. By acknowledging and understanding the diversity of experiences within the BDSM community, we can develop more nuanced and effective approaches to supporting individuals who engage in these practices.

It is also important to recognize that the connection between BDSM and mental health is complex and multifaceted. While healthy BDSM practices can have many potential benefits for mental health, they are not a panacea or a substitute for professional mental health care. Individuals who engage in BDSM should be encouraged to seek out appropriate mental health support as needed, and mental health professionals should be trained to understand the unique needs and experiences of those who engage in BDSM.

Finally, as our understanding of BDSM and mental health continues to evolve, it is important to remain open to new ideas and perspectives. The BDSM community is constantly evolving and changing, and our understanding of mental health is similarly dynamic. By remaining open to new perspectives and ideas, we can continue to explore the potential benefits and risks of BDSM practices for mental health, and develop more effective interventions and support services for those who engage in them.

We understand that our exploration of the connection between BDSM and mental health is far from complete. While we have made great strides in understanding the potential benefits of healthy BDSM practices for mental health, there is still much to be explored and understood. By continuing to conduct research, acknowledge the diversity of experiences within the BDSM community, remain open to new ideas and perspectives, and encourage individuals who engage in BDSM to seek out appropriate mental health support, we can continue to promote mental health and well-being for all.

References

Baker, A. C. (2016). Sacred kink: finding psychological meaning at the intersection of BDSM and spiritual experience. *Sexual and Relationship Therapy*, *33*(4), 440–453. https://doi.org/10.1080/14681994.2016.1205185

Baker, A. J. (2019). Consensual slavery: A framework for ethical BDSM. *Journal of Sex Research*, *56*(4 - 5), 597–610. https://doi.org/10.1080/00224499.2018.1483332

Baumeister, R. F. (1988). Masochism as Escape from Self. *The Journal of Sex Research*, *25*(1), 28–59. https://www.jstor.org/stable/3812869

Blizard, R. A. (2001). Masochistic and Sadistic Ego States. *Journal of Trauma & Dissociation*, *2*(4), 37–58. https://doi.org/10.1300/j229v02n04_03

Bloomer, M. L. (2019). Exploring the Framework of Consent and Negotiation in the BDSM Community for Broader Application within Corporate Environments - ProQuest. Www.proquest.com. https://www.proquest.com/openview/13bc385ed2f76ee0f1e5e97c43cb4d88/1?pq-origsite=gscholar&cbl=18750&diss=y

Brown, A., Barker, E. D., & Rahman, Q. (2019). A Systematic Scoping Review of the Prevalence, Etiological, Psychological, and Interpersonal Factors Associated with BDSM. The Journal of Sex Research, 57(6), 781–811. https://doi.org/10.1080/00224499.2019.1665619

Brown, C. C., Morey, L. C., & Lycan, C. (2016). EEG neurofeedback as adjunct to psychotherapy for complex developmental trauma-related disorders: Case study and treatment rationale. Traumatology, 22(3), 153–160. https://doi.org/10.1037/trm0000073

Combridge, K., & Lastella, M. (2023). Stigmatisation of People with Deviant Sexual Interest: A Comparative Study. Sexes, 4(1), 7–25. https://doi.org/10.3390/sexes4010002

Connolly, P. H. (2006). Psychological Functioning of Bondage/Domination/Sado-Masochism (BDSM) Practitioners. Journal of Psychology & Human Sexuality, 18(1), 79–120. https://doi.org/10.1300/j056v18n01_05

Cross, P. A., & Matheson, K. (2006). Understanding Sadomasochism. Journal of Homosexuality, 50(2-3), 133–166. https://doi.org/10.1300/j082v50n02_07

Cutler, B., Lee, E., Cutler, N., & Sagarin, B. (2020). Partner Selection, Power Dynamics, and Mutual Care Giving in Long-Term Self-Defined BDSM Couples. Journal of Positive Sexuality, 6(2), 86–114. https://doi.org/10.51681/1.624

Dahan, O. (2019). Submission, pain and pleasure: Considering an evolutionary hypothesis concerning sexual masochism. Psychology of Consciousness: Theory, Research, and Practice, 6(4), 386–403. https://doi.org/10.1037/cns0000202

Dancer, P. L., Kleinplatz, P. J., & Moser, C. (2006). 24/7 SM Slavery. Journal of Homosexuality, 50(2-3), 81–101. https://doi.org/10.1300/j082v50n02_05

Echterdiek, F., Kitterer, D., Schwenger, V., & Latus, J. (2018). Severe acute kidney injury due to violent sadomasochistic play. BMJ Case Reports, bcr-2018-224813. https://doi.org/10.1136/bcr-2018-224813

Fan, Y., & Han, S. (2008). Temporal dynamic of neural mechanisms involved in empathy for pain: An event-related brain potential study. Neuropsychologia, 46(1), 160–173. https://doi.org/10.1016/j.neuropsychologia.2007.07.023

Fuentes, S. (2019). Caring about Aftercare: Thesis Presentation of Initial Findings. https://doi.org/10.15760/honors.837

Gunning, J. N., Rubinsky, V., Aragón, A., Roldán, M., McMahon, T., & Cooke-Jackson, A. (2023). A Preliminary Investigation into Intersections of Sexual Communication in Bondage, Domination, Sadomasochism and Disability. Sexuality & Culture, 1–17. https://doi.org/10.1007/s12119-022-10058-8

Hansen-Brown, A. A., & Jefferson, S. E. (2022). Perceptions of and stigma toward BDSM practitioners. Current Psychology, 1–9. https://doi.org/10.1007/s12144-022-03112-z

Hansen-Brown, A. T., & Jefferson, K. (2022). Understanding attitudes toward BDSM: The role of social dominance orientation, authoritarianism, and traditional gender roles. Journal of Homosexuality, 69(2), 131–146.

Hawkin, M. J., & O'Hare, T. (2017). Exploring the impact of BDSM on interpersonal functioning: A qualitative phenomenological study. Archives of Sexual Behavior, 46(2), 435–446. https://doi.org/10.1007/s10508-016-0764-9

Hawkin, R., & Hawkin, R., & O'Hare, T. (2017). BDSM as therapy? An exploration of submissive headspace, T. (2017). BDSM as therapy? An exploration of submissive headspace. Archives of Sexual Behavior, 46(1), 219–235.

Hébert, A., & Weaver, A. (2014). BDSM: A subcultural analysis of sacrifices and delights. Deviant Behavior, 35(2), 144–162. https://doi.org/10.1080/01639625.2013.834145

Hébert, A., & Weaver, A. (2014). Bondage and discipline, dominance and submission, and sadomasochism (BDSM) from an integrative biopsychosocial perspective: A systematic review. The Journal of Sex Research, 51(4), 367–378. https://doi.org/10.1080/00224499.2012.719167

Hébert, A., & Weaver, A. (2015). Perks, problems, and the people who play: A qualitative exploration of dominant and submissive BDSM roles. The Canadian Journal of Human Sexuality, 24(1), 49–62. https://doi.org/10.3138/cjhs.2467

Hillier, K. (2019). ScholarWorks The Impact of Childhood Trauma and Personality on Kinkiness in Adulthood. https://core.ac.uk/download/pdf/217233885.pdf

Kleinplatz, P. J. (2006). Learning from Extraordinary Lovers. Journal of Homosexuality, 50(2-3), 325–348. https://doi.org/10.1300/j082v50n02_16

Kleinplatz, P. J., & Moser, C. (2006). The politics of BDSM: Autonomy, informed consent, and the feminist debate. Journal of Homosexuality, 50(2-3), 21–49. https://doi.org/10.1300/j082v50n02_02

Kleinplatz, P. J., & Moser, C. (2006). The therapeutic value of BDSM. Journal of Homosexuality, 50(2-3), 301–315. https://doi.org/10.1300/j082v50n02_14

Kleinplatz, P. J., & Moser, C. (2014). Sadomasochism - Powerful Pleasures (P. J. Kleinplatz & C. Moser, Eds.). Routledge. https://doi.org/10.4324/9781315801582

Klement, K. R., Lee, E. M., Ambler, J. K., Hanson, S. A., Comber, E., Wietting, D., Wagner, M. F., Burns, V. R., Cutler, B., Cutler, N., Reid, E., & Sagarin, B. J. (2016). Extreme rituals in a BDSM context: the physiological and psychological effects of the "Dance of Souls." Culture, Health & Sexuality, 19(4), 453–469. https://doi.org/10.1080/13691058.2016.1234648

Klement, K. R., Sagarin, B. J., & Lee, E. M. (2016). Participating in a Culture of Consent May Be Associated With Lower Rape-Supportive Beliefs. The Journal of Sex Research, 54(1), 130–134. https://doi.org/10.1080/00224499.2016.1168353

Kolmes, K., Stock, W., & Moser, C. (2006). Investigating bias in psychotherapy with BDSM clients. Journal of Homosexuality, 50(2-3), 301–324. https://doi.org/10.1300/j082v50n02_16

Mikulincer, M., & Shaver, P. R. (2016). Attachment in Adulthood, Second Edition: Structure, Dynamics, and Change. Https://Www.routledge.com/Attachment-In-Adulthood-Second-Edition-Structure-Dynamics-And-Change/Mikulincer-Shaver/P/Book/9781462533817; Routledge & CRC Press. https://www.routledge.com/Attachment-in-Adulthood-Second-Edition-Structure-Dynamics-and-Change/Mikulincer-Shaver/p/book/9781462533817

Moser, C. (2010). Demystifying therapy for clients: A primer of BDSM-informed psychotherapy. Journal of Homosexuality, 57(3), 303–320. https://doi.org/10.1080/00918369.2010.486241

Moser, C., & Kleinplatz, P. J. (2006). DSM-IV-TRand the Paraphilias. Journal of Psychology & Human Sexuality, 17(3-4), 91–109. https://doi.org/10.1300/j056v17n03_05

Moser, C., & Kleinplatz, P. J. (2006). Introduction. Journal of Homosexuality, 50(2-3), 1–15. https://doi.org/10.1300/j082v50n02_01

New, C. M., Batchelor, L. C., Schimmel-Bristow, A., Schaeffer-Smith, M., Magsam, E., Bridges, S. K., Brown, E. L., & McKenzie, T. (2021). In their own words: getting it right for kink clients. Sexual and Relationship Therapy, 1–19. https://doi.org/10.1080/14681994.2021.1965112

Pietrusza, C. (2019). Duquesne Scholarship Collection Electronic Theses and Dissertations Kink in Flux: BDSM theory and sexual praxis. https://dsc.duq.edu/cgi/viewcontent.cgi?article=2810&context=etd

Pincus, A. L., Choate, L. H., Gurtman, M. B., Johnson, W., Lynam, D. R., Swann, W. B., & Wright, A. G. (2018). The power and promise of process-oriented approaches in psychological science. Psychological Science, 29(3), 307–318. https://doi.org/10.1177/0956797617738696

Price, M., Thompson, R., & D'Andrea, W. (2019). Integration of cognitive behavioral therapy for insomnia. Journal of Psychotherapy Integration, 29(3), 263–280. https://doi.org/10.1037/int0000133

Ramey, M. (2013). Exploring power exchange dynamics in BDSM. Exploring Power Exchange Dynamics in BDSM., 2(2), 22–27. https://doi.org/10.6084/m9.figshare.661583.v1

Richters, J., De Visser, R. O., Rissel, C. E., Grulich, A. E., & Smith, A. M. A. (2008). Demographic and Psychosocial Features of Participants in Bondage and Discipline, "Sadomasochism" or Dominance and Submission (BDSM): Data from a National Survey. The Journal of Sexual Medicine, 5(7), 1660–1668. https://doi.org/10.1111/j.1743-6109.2008.00795.x

Sagarin, B. J., Cutler, B., Cutler, N., Lawler-Sagarin, K. A., & Matuszewich, L. (2008). Hormonal Changes and Couple Bonding in Consensual Sadomasochistic Activity. Archives of Sexual Behavior, 38(2), 186–200. https://doi.org/10.1007/s10508-008-9374-5

Schori, A., Jackowski, C., & Schön, C. A. (2021). How safe is BDSM? A literature review on fatal outcome in BDSM play. International Journal of Legal Medicine, 136(1). https://doi.org/10.1007/s00414-021-02674-0

Schuerwegen, A., Morrens, M., Wuyts, E., Huys, W., Goethals, K., & De Zeeuw-Jans, I. (2022). The psychology of kink: A survey study investigating stigma and psychological mechanisms in BDSM. European Psychiatry, 65(S1), S804–S804. https://doi.org/10.1192/j.eurpsy.2022.2079

Simula, B. L. (2019). Pleasure, power, and pain: A review of the literature on the experiences of BDSM participants. Sociology Compass, 13(3), e12668. https://doi.org/10.1111/soc4.12668

Simula, B. L. (2021). Introduction to the special issue: BDSM Studies. Sexualities, 24(5-6), 136346072199303. https://doi.org/10.1177/1363460721993039

Steele, K., & van der Hart, O. (2015). Working with dissociation in traumatized children and adolescents: An integrative approach. Journal of Child & Adolescent Trauma, 8(4), 275–286. https://doi.org/10.1007/s40653-015-0061-7

Ten Brink, S., Coppens, V., Huys, W., & Morrens, M. (2020). The Psychology of Kink: a Survey Study into the Relationships of Trauma and Attachment Style with BDSM Interests. Sexuality Research and Social Policy, 18(1), 1–12. https://doi.org/10.1007/s13178-020-00438-w

Turley, E. L. (2022). Unperverting the perverse: Sacrificing transgression for normalised acceptance in the BDSM subculture. Sexualities, 136346072211327. https://doi.org/10.1177/13634607221132727

Turley, E. L., King, N., & Monro, S. (2018). "You want to be swept up in it all": illuminating the erotic in BDSM. Psychology & Sexuality, 9(2), 148–160. https://doi.org/10.1080/19419899.2018.1448297

Waters, J. A., & Galupo, M. P. (2019). The impact of consensual sadomasochistic practices on the psychological well-being of practitioners: A systematic review. Psychology of Sexual Orientation and Gender Diversity, 6(1), 3–17. https://doi.org/10.1037/sgd0000329

Weinberg, M. S., Williams, C. J., & Moser, C. (1984). The Social Constituents of Sadomasochism. Social Problems, 31(4), 379–389. https://doi.org/10.2307/800385

Weiss, M. D. (2006). BDSM Basics for Beginners - A Guide for Dominants and Submissives Starting to Explore the Lifestyle: 9781300837107: Fegatofi, Michelle: Libros. Greenery Press.

Williams, DJ., Prior, E. E., Alvarado, T., Thomas, J. N., & Christensen, M. C. (2016). Is Bondage and Discipline, Dominance and Submission, and Sadomasochism Recreational Leisure? A Descriptive Exploratory Investigation. The Journal of Sexual Medicine, 13(7), 1091–1094. https://doi.org/10.1016/j.jsxm.2016.05.001

Wismeijer, A. A. J., & van Assen, M. A. L. M. (2013). Psychological Characteristics of BDSM Practitioners. The Journal of Sexual Medicine, 10(8), 1943–1952. https://doi.org/10.1111/jsm.12192

Wuyts, E., De Neef, N., Coppens, V., Fransen, E., Schellens, E., Van Der Pol, M., & Morrens, M. (2020). Between Pleasure and Pain: A Pilot Study on the Biological Mechanisms Associated With BDSM Interactions in Dominants and Submissives. The Journal of Sexual Medicine, 17(4), 784–792. https://doi.org/10.1016/j.jsxm.2020.01.001

Wuyts, E., & Morrens, M. (2022). The Biology of BDSM: A Systematic Review. The Journal of Sexual Medicine, 19(1), 144–157. https://doi.org/10.1016/j.jsxm.2021.11.002

Yost, M. R., & Hunter, L. E. (2012). BDSM practitioners' understandings of their initial attraction to BDSM sexuality: essentialist and constructionist narratives. Psychology and Sexuality, 3(3), 244–259. https://doi.org/10.1080/19419899.2012.700028

About the Author

Chris Cornejo is a psychotherapist with over 20 years of experience in the BDSM community. His passion for BDSM and knowledge of psychology have led him to write his first book, exploring the connection between BDSM and mental health.

As a psychotherapist, Chris has worked with clients from the military and BDSM communities, and his personal experiences with BDSM have allowed him to appreciate the nuances of the lifestyle and understand the different motivations behind kink exploration.

Chris has written hundreds of articles on the intersection of psychology and BDSM, with many of them on his website and social media. He also hosts a podcast called The Kink Perspective, which delves into the psychological aspects of BDSM.

While Chris plans to continue writing and exploring the connections between BDSM and mental health, he remains committed to his psychotherapy practice and giving back to the BDSM community, with potential plans to write more books in the future.